Arterial Blood Gas Analysis
making it easy

Full the full range of M&K Publishing books please visit our website:

www.mkupdate.co.uk

Arterial Blood Gas Analysis
making it easy
• • •
Anne McLeod

Arterial blood gas analysis – making it easy

Anne McLeod

ISBN: 9781910451-05-2

First published 2016

All rights reserved. No part of this publication may be reproduced, stored in a retrieval system, or transmitted in any form or by any means, electronic, mechanical, photocopying, recording or otherwise, without either the prior permission of the publishers or a licence permitting restricted copying in the United Kingdom issued by the Copyright Licensing Agency, 90 Tottenham Court Road, London, W1T 4LP. Permissions may be sought directly from M&K Publishing, phone: 01768 773030, fax: 01768 781099 or email: publishing@mkupdate.co.uk

Any person who does any unauthorised act in relation to this publication may be liable to criminal prosecution and civil claims for damages.

British Library Cataloguing in Publication Data
A catalogue record for this book is available from the British Library

Notice

Clinical practice and medical knowledge constantly evolve. Standard safety precautions must be followed, but, as knowledge is broadened by research, changes in practice, treatment and drug therapy may become necessary or appropriate. Readers must check the most current product information provided by the manufacturer of each drug to be administered and verify the dosages and correct administration, as well as contraindications. It is the responsibility of the practitioner, utilising the experience and knowledge of the patient, to determine dosages and the best treatment for each individual patient. Any brands mentioned in this book are as examples only and are not endorsed by the publisher. Neither the publisher nor the authors assume any liability for any injury and/or damage to persons or property arising from this publication.

Disclaimer

M&K Publishing cannot accept responsibility for the contents of any linked website or online resource. The existence of a link does not imply any endorsement or recommendation of the organisation or the information or views which may be expressed in any linked website or online resource. We cannot guarantee that these links will operate consistently and we have no control over the availability of linked pages.

To contact M&K Publishing write to:
M&K Update Ltd · The Old Bakery · St. John's Street
Keswick · Cumbria CA12 5AS
Tel: 01768 773030 · Fax: 01768 781099
publishing@mkupdate.co.uk
www.mkupdate.co.uk

Designed and typeset by Mary Blood
Printed in England by McKanes, Keswick

Contents

List of illustrations vi

List of tables vii

About the author viii

Introduction ix

Acknowledgements x

Chapter 1 1
What are arterial blood gases?

Chapter 2 5
Respiratory gases

Chapter 3 15
Acid-base balance

Chapter 4 23
Interpreting blood gases

Chapter 5 31
How to respond to the results

Chapter 6 41
Caring for a patient with an arterial line

Quiz answers 49

References 61

Index 62

List of illustrations

Figure 2.1   Pulmonary ventilation 6

Figure 2.2   External respiration 7

Figure 2.3   Internal respiration 8

Figure 2.4   Oxygen–haemoglobin dissociation curve 9

Figure 2.5   Effect of pH on oxygen dissociation curve 10

Figure 2.6   Effect of temperature on oxygen dissociation 11

Figure 2.7   Carbon dioxide transport (cells–blood) 12

Figure 2.8   Carbon dioxide transport (blood to alveoli) 12

Figure 3.1   Primary active secretion of hydrogen 19

Figure 3.2   Secondary active transport of hydrogen 20

Figure 4.1   Steps in interpreting blood gases 26

Figure 6.1   The patient's hand before starting an Allen's test 42

Figure 6.2   Blanching of the palm during occlusion of the ulnar and radial arteries 42

Figure 6.3   Flushing of the palm after the ulnar artery has been released, demonstrating good collateral circulation 43

Figure 6.4   Arterial line dressing 45

Figure 6.5   Correct arterial line set-up 45

Figure 6.6   Normal arterial waveform 46

Figure 6.7   Underdamp arterial waveform 47

Figure 6.8   Overdamp arterial waveform 47

List of tables

Table 4.1   Causes of respiratory disturbances in arterial blood gases 23

Table 4.2   Causes of metabolic disturbances in arterial blood gases 24

Table 4.3   Interpretation of arterial blood gases 27

Table 5.1   Actions to take to resolve changes in arterial blood gases 35

About the author

Anne McLeod is a Senior Lecturer in Critical Care at the School of Health Sciences, City University, London.

Introduction

Arterial blood gases are frequently assessed in critical care or if a patient deteriorates unexpectedly. Analysing these blood gases helps practitioners to identify key physiological changes as well as finding out whether interventions are appropriate or need adjusting. However, many practitioners are uncertain how to interpret blood gases and what actions should be taken when alterations have been identified.

This book offers an opportunity to develop knowledge and skill in this core aspect of assessing critically ill adult patients. Key physiology (such as the carriage of respiratory gases) is incorporated and applied to the parameters measured in blood gas analysis. Respiratory and metabolic causes of alterations in blood gases are also explored and explained in relation to possible changes in blood gases. A step-by-step guide to assessing blood gases is provided, and examples of blood gases have been included for interpretation.

To develop knowledge further, case studies have been included in Chapter 5 to demonstrate how patient care (and the changing patient situation) can be positively influenced by correct interpretation of blood gases. Quizzes (using a question and short answer format) are provided so that you can test yourself as you work through the book.

Note: Arterial oxygen/carbon dioxide measurements are referred to as PaO_2 or $PaCO_2$. Tissue or cellular oxygen/carbon dioxide has been referred to as pO_2 or pCO_2. The unit of measurement used is kPa; to convert to mmHg, please multiply by 7.5.

Acknowledgements

Many thanks to Steve for his feedback and suggestions.

1

What are arterial blood gases?

Interpreting arterial blood gases (ABGs) is a key skill for critical care practitioners, as these results provide important information about the patient's current condition, what interventions are required, and whether the patient is responding to treatment. ABGs offer accurate and thorough information about the body's ability to maintain an environment that is suitable for cellular activity and function. Changes in metabolic and/or respiratory function are reflected in the parameters measured and the body's ability to maintain a normal acid-base balance.

Five key parameters are measured:
- The pH
- Oxygen
- Carbon dioxide
- Bicarbonate
- Base excess.

The pH

The pH reflects the body's internal environment and its ability to maintain the balance between acidotic and alkalotic substances. The pH indicates the hydrogen concentration within the body, which is influenced by both respiratory gases and solutes (such as sodium, chloride, potassium and bicarbonate) within the blood. The hydrogen ion concentration of extracellular fluid is closely regulated, as hydrogen concentration influences cellular function such as enzyme reactions.

The normal pH is 7.35–7.45, and ideally 7.4 (Adam & Osborne 2005). When loss of hydrogen exceeds gain, the arterial plasma concentration of hydrogen goes down (the pH goes above 7.4) and the condition is called alkalosis. When gain exceeds loss, the concentration increases and the pH drops, leading to acidosis. A pH that is less than 7.35 is acidosis, and one that is more than 7.45 is alkalosis.

Oxygen

The partial pressure of oxygen (PaO_2) within the arterial blood reflects the amount of oxygen in the blood, and can therefore offer information about hypoxaemia. The PaO_2 will be influenced by how well oxygen can diffuse into the blood from the alveoli.

A normal PaO_2 is 10–13.3kPa (Adam & Osborne 2005).

Carbon dioxide

The partial pressure of carbon dioxide ($PaCO_2$) is an important parameter obtained during blood gas analysis. $PaCO_2$ is largely influenced by the ventilatory function of the respiratory system and is therefore dependent on the mechanics of breathing.

A normal $PaCO_2$ is 4.6–6kPa (Adam & Osborne, 2005).

Bicarbonate

Bicarbonate (HCO_3^-) is alkaline and is vital in the pH buffering system to maintain a stable acid-base balance. The loss of bicarbonate has a similar impact to gaining hydrogen ions, whereas gaining bicarbonate has virtually the same net effect as losing hydrogen.

A normal HCO_3^- is 22–26mmol/l (Adam & Osborne 2005).

Base excess (BE)

An important element of acid-base balance is the measurement of base excess (BE). BE is the amount of strong acid required to titrate blood to a pH of 7.40 when the patient's temperature is 37°C and there is a $PaCO_2$ of 5.3kPa. A base deficit (negative number) indicates the amount of strong base that needs to be added to each litre of blood to return the pH to 7.4, whereas a base excess (positive reading) suggests the amount of strong acid that must be added to each litre of blood to achieve a pH of 7.4. Base excess indicates the amount of available buffer that is present. Buffers are an important part of maintaining a normal pH, as buffers reversibly bind hydrogen ions. This helps to control the amount of hydrogen within the blood and therefore the pH.

A normal BE range is from -2 to +2 (Adam and Osborne, 2005).

Other readings

Blood gas analysers also measure other solutes within the blood, such as sodium, potassium and glucose. Information about haemoglobin (Hb) and haemocrit is usually obtained as well. All these results give practitioners information about key changes that may require further investigation.

Some blood gas analysers will give readings of pO_2 and pCO_2 in mmHG rather than kPa. To convert mmHg into kPa, divide the number by 7.5. To convert kPa into mmHg, multiply the number by 7.5.

Test yourself

1. What are normal blood gas values?
2. Which ion is measured by pH?
3. What term is used if the PaO_2 is below normal range?
4. Which aspect of respiratory physiology affects $PaCO_2$?
5. Is bicarbonate an acid or alkaline substance?
6. How do buffers help to control pH?

2

Respiratory gases

Arterial blood gases offer useful information on the functioning of the respiratory system. This chapter will consider the physiological processes involved in gas exchange, oxygen delivery and excretion of carbon dioxide.

Respiratory physiology
There are three main processes involved in gas exchange:
1. Pulmonary ventilation
2. External respiration
3. Internal respiration.

1 Pulmonary ventilation ('breathing')
In this process, respiratory gases are exchanged between the atmosphere and the lungs. This happens when a pressure gradient exists between the lungs and the atmosphere.

Inspiration
Inspiration takes place when the pressure in the lungs is lower than atmospheric pressure. The reduction in pressure occurs when the volume of the lungs increases; this is achieved through contraction of the respiratory muscles and is explained by Boyle's law. Boyle's law states that if the volume of a closed container increases, the pressure inside the container reduces, and vice versa when the volume of the container becomes smaller (Tortora & Derrickson 2009).

The main respiratory muscle is the diaphragm, which is innervated by the phrenic nerve. When the diaphragm contracts, it changes from its resting domed shape to a flattened position, and the vertical diameter of the thoracic cavity increases. This action accounts for the movement of more than two-thirds of the air that enters the lungs during inspiration (Tortora & Derrickson 2009). In conjunction with the diaphragm, contraction of the external intercostal muscles lifts the ribs up and out, thus increasing the anterior–posterior diameter of the thorax.

Arterial Blood Gas Analysis – making it easy

The contraction of the respiratory muscles leads to a reduction in the pressure inside the lungs, as per Boyle's law. The intra-alveolar pressure drops from 760mmHg to 758mmHg. This leads to a pressure gradient between atmospheric pressure and intra-alveolar pressure, as the atmospheric pressure is 760mmHg. This pressure gradient allows air to enter the lungs and inspiration to occur. Air continues to enter until the pressures equalise.

At rest, the intrapleural pressures are slightly sub-atmospheric, with a pressure of 756mmHg prior to inspiration. However, during inspiration, the intrapleural pressure reduces to 754mmHg. This creates a vacuum effect, with the walls of the lungs being sucked outwards, further aiding expansion of the lungs.

Expiration

Expiration is also achieved through changes in pressure gradients, but the pressure inside the lungs becomes greater than atmospheric pressure. This occurs as a result of relaxation of the respiratory muscles, which returns them to their resting position. Therefore, the diaphragm relaxes and becomes dome-shaped, while relaxation of the intercostal muscles drops the ribs down and inwards. This relaxation is passive and leads to a reduction in the volume of the lungs. This, in turn, increases the intra-alveolar pressure, leading to expiration, in which air moves out of the lungs (see Figure 2.1).

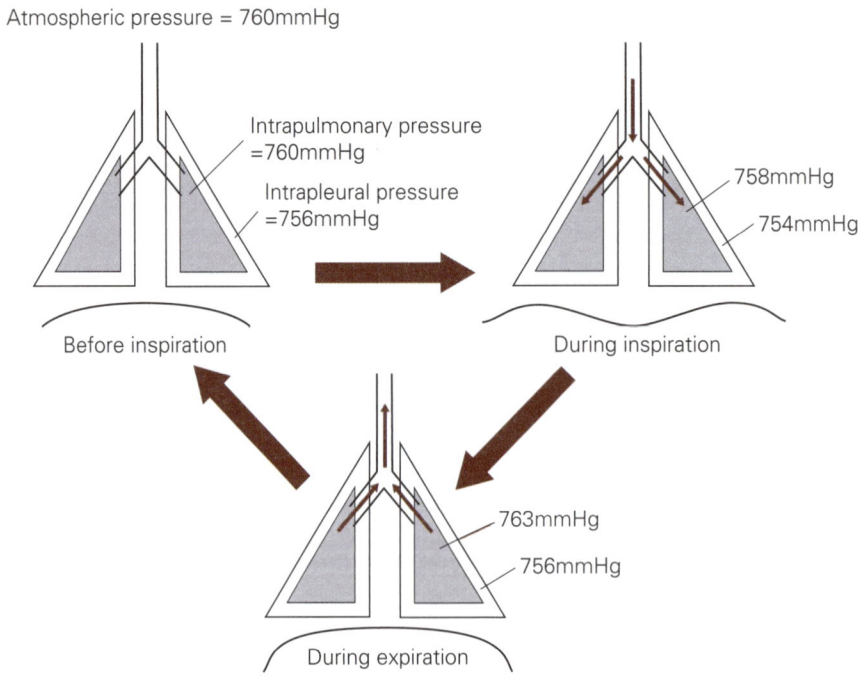

Figure 2.1 Pulmonary ventilation

2 External respiration

External respiration refers to the diffusion of respiratory gases between the alveoli and the blood. It leads to the reoxygenation of deoxygenated blood, which had returned to the lungs. Diffusion is the movement of a molecule from a high to a low concentration, to make the concentrations equal. As respiratory gases are soluble in lipids, they easily pass across cell membranes by diffusion.

Blood returning to the heart from the systemic circulation has a PaO_2 of 40mmHg (5.33kPa) and a $PaCO_2$ of 45mmHg (6kPa). However, in the alveoli, there is a pO_2 of 105mmHg (14kPa) and a pCO_2 of 40mmHg (5.33kPa). Therefore, a concentration gradient exists between the alveoli and the blood, which leads to oxygen diffusing into the blood and carbon dioxide diffusing into the alveoli. This continues until the concentration gradients equalise, with the result that the blood leaving the lungs is oxygenated and carbon dioxide is expired during exhalation (Vander *et al.* 2003) (see Figure 2.2).

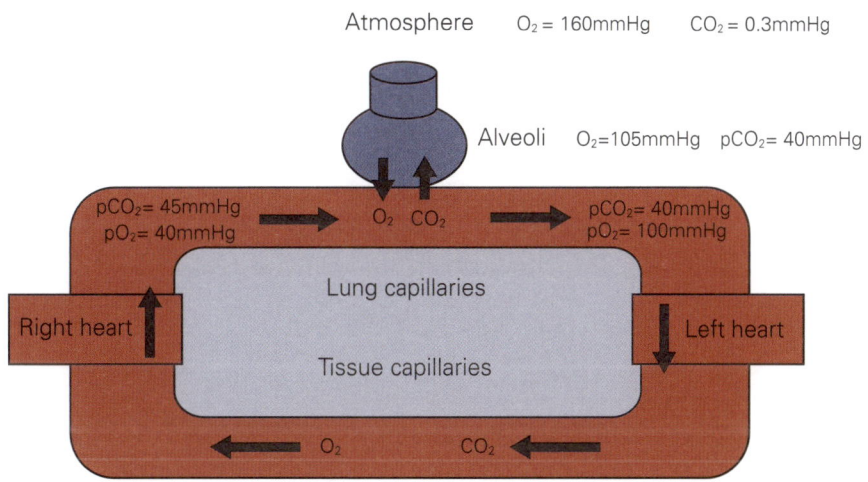

Figure 2.2 External respiration

There are several features of the lungs that enhance external respiration. Firstly, the alveoli–capillary membrane is only 0.5μm thick. (If the membrane were thicker or became thickened due to illness, diffusion would be impaired.) In addition, respiratory gases are lipid soluble, which means they can easily diffuse through the cell membranes. Secondly, there is a very large surface area, across which diffusion can occur. There are around 300 million alveoli within the lungs, which creates a 70m² surface area. Each alveolus is surrounded by a capillary network, which ensures that there is a good blood supply to enable effective gas exchange, with approximately 900ml of blood participating in gas exchange at any one time. Finally, the pulmonary capillaries are very narrow, which means that the red blood cells flow through the capillaries in single file. This allows for the maximum perfusion, as each red blood cell can participate in gas exchange (Tortora & Derrickson 2009).

3 Internal respiration

Internal respiration is the exchange of gases between the blood and the cells. During external respiration, blood is reoxygenated so the blood leaving the left ventricle has a PaO_2 of 100mmHg (13.3kPa) and a $PaCO_2$ of 40mmHg (5.33kPa). Gas diffusion occurs between the blood and the body's cells, as the cells have a pO_2 of 40mmHg (5.33kPa) and a pCO_2 of 45mmHg (6kPa). Because there is a concentration gradient, oxygen diffuses into the tissues and carbon dioxide diffuses into the blood. Therefore, the blood returning back to the heart has a PaO_2 of 40mmHg (5.33kPa) and a $PaCO_2$ of 45mmHg (6kPa), and the cycle of external and internal respiration restarts (see Figure 2.3).

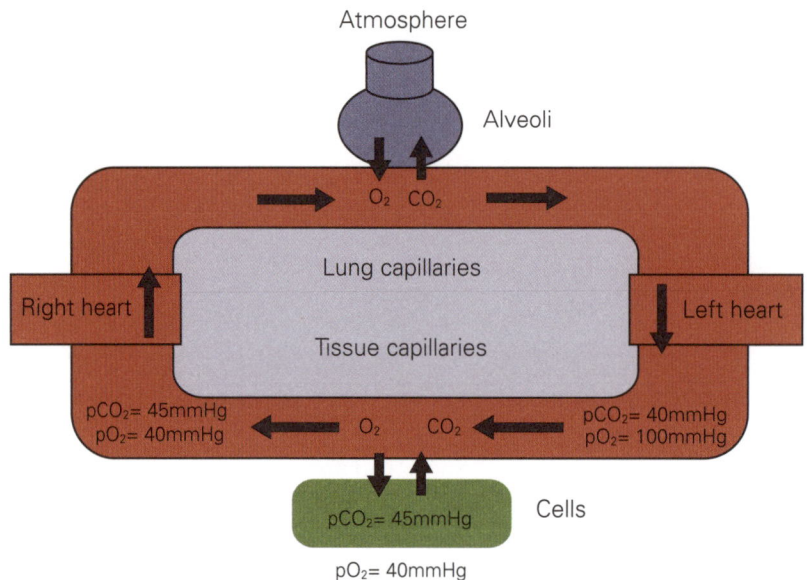

Figure 2.3 Internal respiration

Transport of gases

The lungs facilitate the oxygenation of blood and excretion of carbon dioxide, while the cardiovascular system is responsible for delivering and removing respiratory gases. Both systems need to be functioning well to ensure good oxygen delivery to tissues, resulting in good tissue perfusion.

Oxygen

Oxygen does not easily dissolve in water. This means that the majority of oxygen (97%) is transported around the body having combined with the haem portion of haemoglobin. The remaining 3% becomes dissolved in plasma. At rest, 100ml of blood contains about 20ml of oxygen (Tortora & Derrickson, 2009). Haemoglobin is made up of haem (which is the red pigment) and globin (which is a protein). The haem portion contains four atoms of iron, each of which can combine with oxygen. This reaction is easily reversible and leads to oxyhaemoglobin forming.

The most important influence in deciding how much oxygen combines with haemoglobin is the pO_2. Full saturation means that all the haemoglobin has been converted to oxyhaemoglobin. If the haemoglobin consists of both haemoglobin and oxyhaemoglobin, then partial saturation is present. The degree of haemoglobin saturation as pO_2 changes is illustrated by the oxygen dissociation curve (see Figure 2.4).

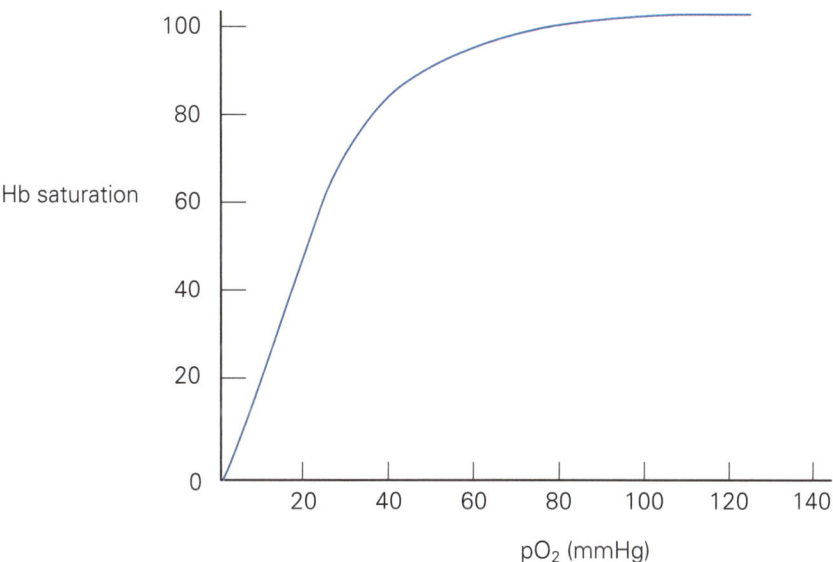

Figure 2.4 Oxygen–haemoglobin dissociation curve

This shows that when the pO_2 is high, there is high affinity of haemoglobin with oxygen, allowing oxygen to bind easily with haemoglobin. This means that the haemoglobin is almost totally saturated. However, when the pO_2 is low, oxygen disassociates from the haemoglobin and becomes available for tissue use. This results in the haemoglobin becoming only partially saturated. Therefore in the pulmonary capillaries, where the pO_2 is high, lots of oxygen binds with haemoglobin. Meanwhile, in the tissues, where the pO_2 is lower, oxygen is released for diffusion.

Arterial Blood Gas Analysis – making it easy

The ability of oxygen to bind with haemoglobin and to be released for use can also be influenced by:

- the pH
- the temperature
- 2,3-diphosphoglycerate (DPG).

The pH

In an acidic environment, oxygen disassociates from haemoglobin more easily: this is known as the Bohr effect (Vander *et al.* 2003). Therefore in situations when tissues are releasing lactic acid and/or a high pCO_2 is present, an acidosis can develop leading to an increase in the amount of oxygen dissociating from haemoglobin (see Figure 2.5).

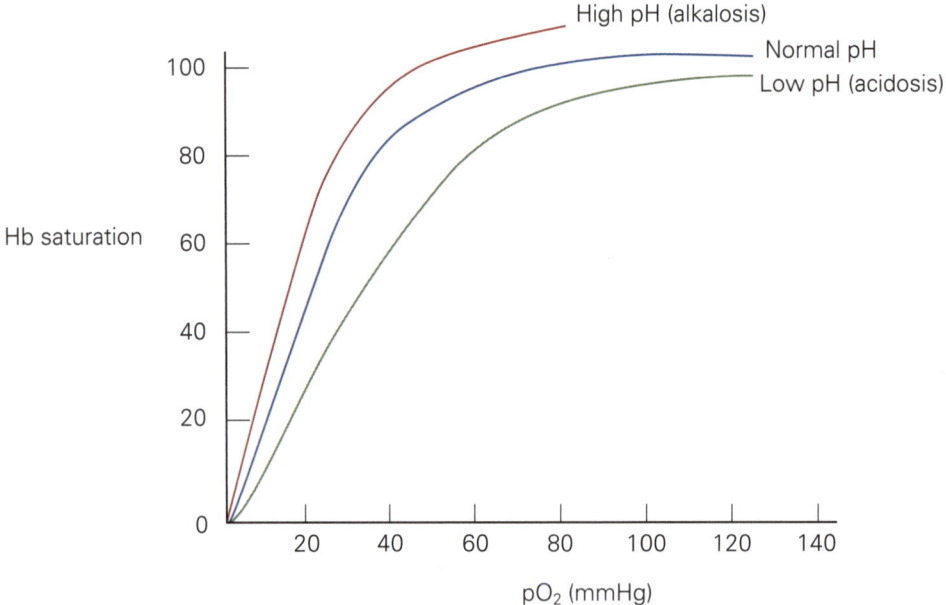

Figure 2.5 Effect of pH on oxygen dissociation curve

The temperature

An increase in temperature leads to more oxygen splitting from haemoglobin. When there is an increase in cellular activity, the heat generated due to the increase in metabolic rate will increase the amount of oxygen released from haemoglobin. This is useful, as the increase in cellular activity increases the oxygen requirements of the cell (see Figure 2.6).

Respiratory gases

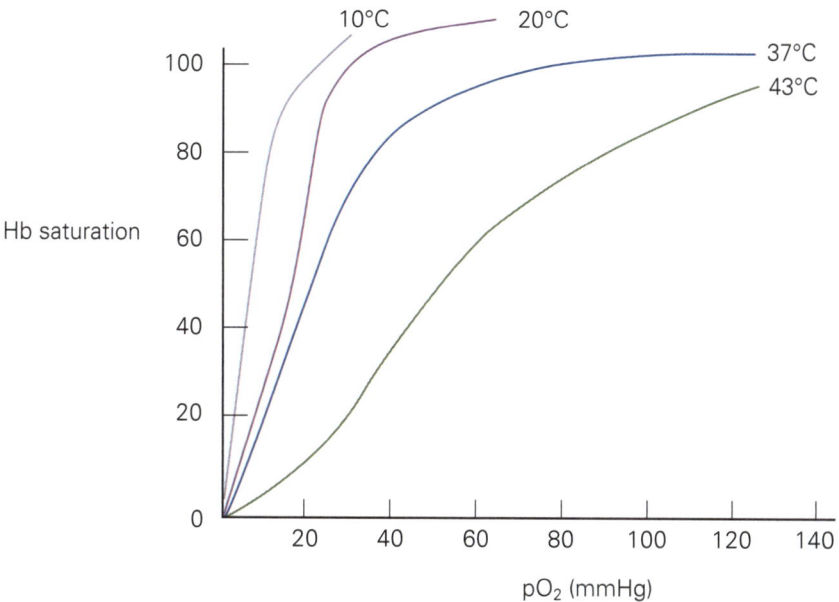

Figure 2.6 Effect of temperature on oxygen dissociation

2,3-diphosphoglycerate (DPG)
DPG is produced during glycolysis and can bind reversibly with haemoglobin, altering its structure to release oxygen. The amount of DPG produced is greatest during times of reduced oxygen delivery to cells. Therefore, DPG enhances tissue oxygenation by helping to maintain the release of oxygen from haemoglobin.

Carbon dioxide
Carbon dioxide is mainly transported around the body within the plasma as bicarbonate (70%). Of the remainder, 23% combines with the globin portion of haemoglobin to form carbaminohaemoglobin, and 7% is dissolved in plasma. The formation of carbaminohaemoglobin is greatly influenced by the pCO_2 and the formation of carbaminohaemoglobin is greatest where the pCO_2 is high (Tortora & Derrickson 2009). Therefore, in the tissues where pCO_2 is high, carbaminohaemoglobin formation is enhanced. Meanwhile, in the lungs, where the pCO_2 is low, CO_2 readily splits from haemoglobin and diffuses into the alveoli.

For the most part, carbon dioxide is transported within the blood as bicarbonate. CO_2 diffuses into the red blood cells, where it reacts with water to form carbonic acid. This reaction requires the enzyme carbonic anhydrase. Carbonic acid then dissociates into hydrogen and bicarbonate. The hydrogen combines with haemoglobin and is therefore buffered. The bicarbonate leaves the red blood cell and enters the plasma.

To maintain the ionic balance of the red blood cell, chloride diffuses from the blood into the red blood cell, where it combines with potassium to form potassium chloride. This is known as the chloride shift (Vander *et al.* 2003). The bicarbonate, which diffused into the plasma, then combines with sodium to form sodium bicarbonate in the blood (see Figure 2.7).

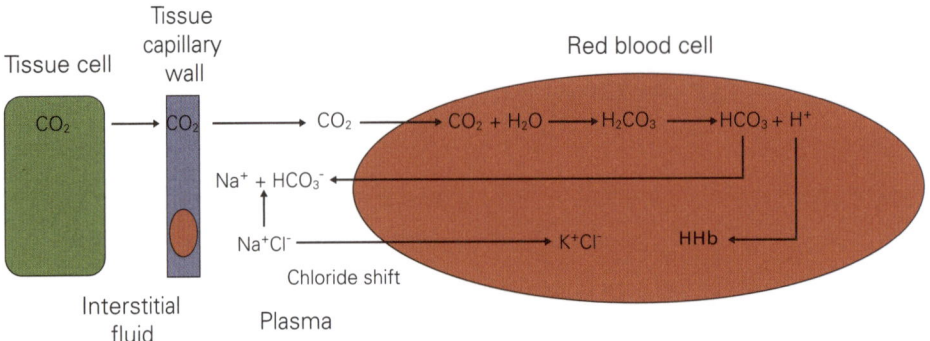

Figure 2.7 Carbon dioxide transport (cells to blood)

Therefore blood returning to the heart contains carbon dioxide that is transported in a variety of forms. In the pulmonary capillaries, the above reactions are reversed. This allows carbon dioxide to diffuse into the alveoli, and it is then excreted during expiration (see Figure 2.8).

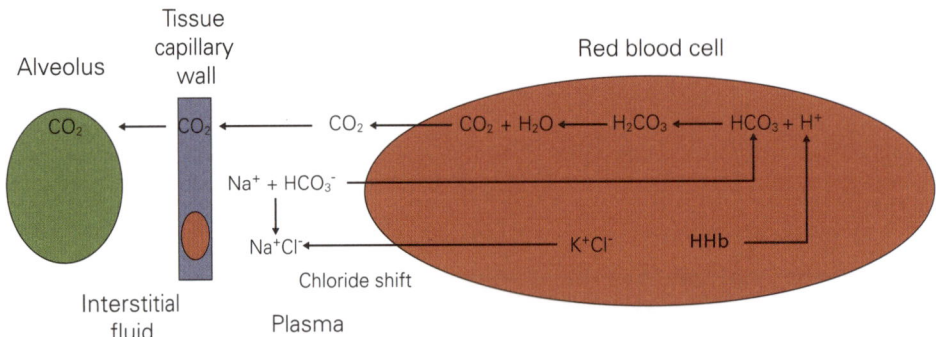

Figure 2.8 Carbon dioxide transport (blood to alveoli)

These processes are key to effective gas exchange, perfusion of tissues and excretion of waste products. The process of carbon dioxide carriage and clearance is also relevant when considering the control of acid-base balance.

Test yourself

1. What are the three key processes involved in gas exchange?
2. What is Boyle's law?
3. In normal respiration, does air enter the lungs under positive or negative pressure?
4. What key features of the alveoli–capillary membrane promote gas exchange?
5. By what process do respiratory gases move between the alveoli and the blood (and vice versa)?
6. What is the main influence for oxygen to disassociate from haemoglobin?
7. How does a decrease in pH affect oxygen disassociation from haemoglobin?
8. What chemical formula illustrates how bicarbonate is formed from carbon dioxide?

3

Acid-base balance

Arterial blood gases offer key information about the body's ability to maintain a balance between acids and bases. Changes in hydrogen concentration can negatively influence nearly all the cellular and bodily functions. The regulation of acid-base balance, and therefore hydrogen ions, involves a number of acid-base buffering systems within the blood, the cells, the lungs and the kidneys. This is important, as careful hydrogen ion regulation is essential for homeostasis and proper functioning of enzyme systems within the body. By ensuring that the concentration of hydrogen normally varies only slightly, these systems prevent any drastic and harmful changes in the hydrogen concentration (and therefore the pH).

What are acids and bases?

Acids are molecules that contain hydrogen atoms, which can be released into solutions. For example, hydrochloric acid (HCl) can ionise in water to form hydrogen (H^+) and chloride (Cl^-). A base is a molecule that can combine with a hydrogen ion. For example, bicarbonate (HCO_3^-) can join with hydrogen to form carbonic acid (H_2CO_3). Proteins are also able to bind hydrogen ions, as some amino acids have a net negative charge that can accept the hydrogen ion. The term 'base' is often used interchangeably with 'alkali'.

Strong and weak acids and bases

Within the body, there are strong and weak acids and bases. These descriptions relate to how quickly or slowly the substance either releases or combines with hydrogen (Tortora & Derrickson 2009). A strong acid is one that rapidly disassociates, releasing large amounts of hydrogen in solution. An example of a strong acid is hydrochloric acid (HCl). Weak acids, such as carbonic acid ($H_2CO_3^-$), release their hydrogen ions more reluctantly.

Likewise, a strong base reacts rapidly and strongly with H^+, facilitating its rapid removal from the solution (Hall 2015). An example of a strong base is hydroxide (OH^-), as it combines with H^+ to form H_2O. Bicarbonate (HCO_3^-) is an example of a weak base, as it binds more weakly with H^+. The weak extracellular acids and bases in extracellular fluid are involved in regulating acid-base balance, with the most important being H_2CO_3 and HCO_3^-.

Normal hydrogen concentration and pH

Hydrogen concentration is usually maintained within tight limits around a normal value of about 0.00004mEq/l (40nEq/L). Variations are normally only about 3–5nEq/L. However, in extreme conditions, the hydrogen ion concentration can vary from as low as 10nEq/L to as high as 160nEq/L without causing death (Hall 2015).

Hydrogen ion concentration is measured on a logarithm scale, using pH units. The pH is inversely related to the hydrogen ion concentration, which means that a low pH indicates a high hydrogen ion concentration. (Conversely, a high pH is a sign of a lower hydrogen concentration.) The normal pH of arterial blood is 7.4, with venous blood having a slightly lower pH (Vander *et al.* 2003).

Control of hydrogen ion concentration

There are three main ways in which hydrogen ion concentration (and therefore pH) is regulated (McGloin & McLeod 2010):

1. The chemical acid-base buffer system avoids excessive changes in hydrogen ion concentration through the immediate combination of hydrogen with buffers. The buffer system works within a fraction of a second of an alteration of hydrogen ion concentration. Buffers can 'store' hydrogen ions until a balance is re-established.
2. The respiratory centre regulates the removal of CO_2 from extracellular fluid. It acts within a few minutes to eliminate CO_2 from the body – this action reduces hydrogen concentration.
3. The kidneys can excrete either acid or alkaline urine, which will influence hydrogen ion concentration. The renal system's response is relatively slow but it is the most powerful of the three acid-base balance regulatory systems.

1 Buffering of hydrogen ions

A buffer is a substance that can reversibly bind hydrogen ions. When the hydrogen ion concentration increases, the ions get bound to an available buffer. If the hydrogen ion concentration decreases, hydrogen ions are released from the buffer. In this way, changes in hydrogen ion concentration are minimised. The bicarbonate buffer system is probably the most important extracellular buffer system, but phosphate and haemoglobin are also important buffers (McGloin & McLeod 2010).

Bicarbonate buffer system

The bicarbonate buffer system consists of a weak acid (H_2CO_3) and a weak base (HCO_3^-). H_2CO_3 is formed in the body by the reaction of CO_2 with H_2O:

$$CO_2 + H_2O \rightleftharpoons H_2CO_3$$

This is a slow reaction and only small amounts of bicarbonate are made, unless the enzyme carbonic anhydrase is present. There are large amounts of carbonic anhydrase in the walls of the alveoli and in the epithelial cells of the renal tubules.

The H_2CO_3 is then ionised to form H^+ and HCO_3^- (Hall 2015):

$$CO_2 + H_2O \rightleftharpoons H_2CO_3 \rightleftharpoons H^+ + HCO_3^-$$

This reaction explains the role of the respiratory and renal systems in maintaining the acid-base balance. These two systems work together to help control the pH but acid-base disturbances will occur when one or both of these control mechanisms becomes impaired. If this happens, the bicarbonate concentration or the pCO_2 of the extracellular fluid will change. 'Metabolic' disturbances will develop if there are changes in the bicarbonate concentration; and 'respiratory' disturbances will develop from changes in the pCO_2 level.

Phosphate buffer system

The phosphate buffer system is not as powerful as the extracellular fluid buffer. However, it contributes to the buffering of renal tubular fluid and intracellular fluids. Dihydrogen phosphate ($H_2PO_4^-$) and hydrogen phosphate (HPO_4^{2-}) are the primary elements used in the phosphate buffer system (Hall 2015). If a strong acid is added to a mixture of these two substances, the hydrogen is accepted by HPO_4^{2-} (base) and is converted to $H_2PO_4^-$. For example, the following occurs when HCl is added to HPO_4^{2-}:

$$HCl + NaHPO_4 \rightarrow NaH_2PO_4 + NaCl$$

Therefore, the strong acid (HCl) is replaced by a weak acid, thus minimising the decrease in pH.

If a strong base is added to the phosphate buffer system, again it will be buffered and replaced by a weaker base, thus minimising the rise in pH (Hall 2015). For example, the following occurs if the strong base OH^- is added to the buffer solution:

$$NaOH + NaH_2PO_4 \rightarrow Na_2HPO_4 + H_2O$$

Proteins as buffers

Proteins are the most plentiful buffer within the body, and help to maintain intracellular pH, which can alter in similar proportions to extracellular fluid pH changes. Although hydrogen and bicarbonate can diffuse through cell membranes, this process occurs in small quantities and can take several hours before there is equilibrium between the intracellular and extracellular concentrations. The exception to this is with red blood cells, as haemoglobin buffers hydrogen, allowing for a rapid equilibrium.

2 Respiratory regulation of acid-base balance

The second way in which the acid-base balance is controlled is by regulating extracellular CO_2. Any increase in ventilation will lead to an increase in CO_2 elimination and a reduction in the hydrogen ion concentration in the extracellular fluid (McGloin & McLeod 2010). Should ventilation reduce, the reverse will happen.

CO_2 is a by-product of cellular metabolism and is continually formed by the body. Changes in either pulmonary ventilation or the rate of cellular CO_2 formation can therefore change the extracellular fluid pCO_2. If the pH of the extracellular fluids is 7.40 with normal alveolar ventilation, doubling the respiratory rate raises the pH to about 7.63. However, a decrease in ventilation to one-fourth of normal reduces the pH by 0.45. If the pH is 7.4 with normal ventilation, a reduction in alveolar ventilation by one-fourth (for example, if the minute volume is 8 litres and it is reduced to 6 litres), will reduce the pH to 6.95 (McGloin and McLeod 2010). This illustrates the extent to which the respiratory system influences the regulation of pH.

At the same time, the pH of extracellular fluid can alter the rate of ventilation. If the pH decreases from a normal value of 7.4 towards 7.0, the alveolar ventilation rate will increase to 4 or 5 times the normal value. Alternatively, if the plasma pH rises above 7.4, a decrease in respiratory rate will be observed (McGloin & McLeod 2010). The change in ventilation rate will lead to a greater change in pH when there is an acidosis, compared with an alkalosis. This is largely due to hypoxaemia developing as the ventilation rate decreases. Conversely, the decrease in PaO_2 will stimulate the respiratory centre to increase the respiratory rate (Hall 2015). Therefore, respiratory compensation for an increase in pH is not effective in normalising pH – in comparison with the response to a decrease in pH.

Nevertheless, if the alteration to the pH has occurred outside the respiratory system, a change in ventilation rate will not be completely effective in returning the hydrogen ion concentration (and therefore pH) back to normal. The respiratory response to an altered hydrogen ion concentration is usually about 50–75% effective. Therefore if the pH falls from 7.4 to 7.0, a respiratory response will return the pH to a value of about 7.2–7.3 (McGloin & McLeod 2010). In some situations (such as when the respiratory system is impaired, due to illness), the sole remaining mechanism to control acid-base balance is the renal response.

Acid-base balance

3 Renal control of acid-base balance

The kidneys have a key role in acid-base balance because they can excrete either acidic or alkaline urine, thus removing either acid or base from the extracellular fluid. Bicarbonate ions are continuously filtered into the renal tubules, which will remove base from the extracellular fluid, as the bicarbonate is then excreted in the urine. However, nearly all the bicarbonate that is filtered is normally reabsorbed back through the tubule, which means that the primary buffer of the body is conserved (McGloin & McLeod 2010). The tubule cells can also secrete hydrogen ions into the filtrate, thus removing acid from the blood. If the hydrogen ions secreted exceed the bicarbonate ions filtered, there will be an overall loss of acid; and the opposite will occur if more bicarbonate ions are filtered than hydrogen ions secreted (Hall 2015).

During an alkalosis, the kidneys do not reabsorb all the filtered bicarbonate, and bicarbonate is lost in urine. This helps to increase the hydrogen ion concentration, thereby returning the pH back towards normal. In acidosis, the kidneys do not excrete bicarbonate. Instead, they reabsorb filtered bicarbonate as well as manufacturing bicarbonate, which enters the bloodstream. This extra bicarbonate again helps to increase the pH, back towards normal.

The kidneys therefore regulate acid-base balance through three fundamental mechanisms:
- Primary active secretion of hydrogen ions
- Secondary secretion of hydrogen ions
- Reabsorption of filtered bicarbonate ions and production of new bicarbonate ions.

Primary active secretion of hydrogen ions

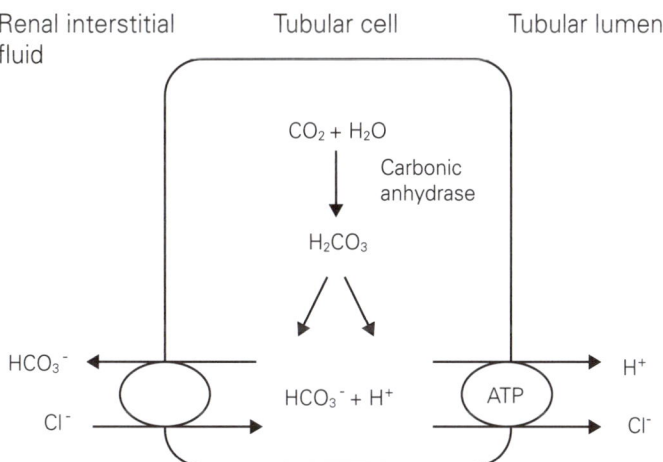

Figure 3.1 Primary active secretion of hydrogen

In the distal convoluted tubule (late portion) and collecting duct of nephrons, the epithelium of the tubule secretes hydrogen by primary active transport. Secretion of hydrogen ions in these cells occurs in two steps. Firstly, dissolved CO_2 combines with H_2O to form H_2CO_3. Secondly, H_2CO_3 disassociates into bicarbonate (which is reabsorbed into blood) and hydrogen (which is secreted into the tubule, using the hydrogen-ATPase mechanism). Although this only accounts for 5% of total hydrogen loss, it is an important mechanism, as maximally acidic urine with a pH of 4.5 is formed (see Figure 3.1).

Secondary secretion of hydrogen ions

The earlier portions of the nephron (proximal convoluted tubule, thick segment of the loop of Henle and early distal convoluted tubule) are able to secrete hydrogen ions into the filtrate by means of a sodium–hydrogen counter-transport mechanism. This secondary active transport of hydrogen is linked to the transport of sodium into the luminal membrane. The movement of hydrogen is against a concentration gradient and requires a sodium–potassium ATPase pump to move sodium across the cell membrane to maintain the concentration gradient (Hall 2015).

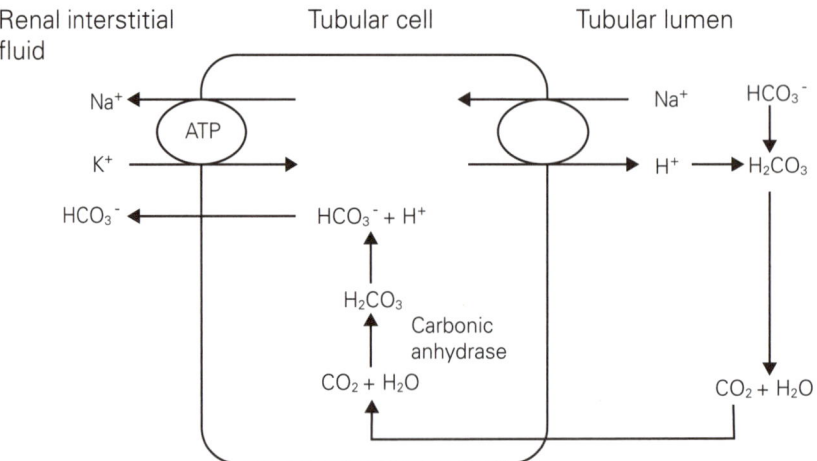

Figure 3.2 Secondary active transport of hydrogen

CO_2 diffuses into the tubular cells or is formed during tubular cellular metabolism. In the presence of carbonic anhydrase, the CO_2 combines with H_2O to form H_2CO_3, which then disassociates into H^+ and HCO_3^-. The hydrogen ions are secreted into the tubular lumen through sodium–hydrogen counter-transport: sodium is carried across the cell membrane by a carrier protein. The hydrogen ion combines with the same carrier protein and is transported out of the cell into filtrate. The bicarbonate ion moves across the cell membrane into the renal interstitial fluid and blood within the peritubular capillaries. Therefore, for every hydrogen ion that is secreted, a bicarbonate ion enters the extracellular fluid (see Figure 3.2).

Reabsorption of filtered bicarbonate ions and production of new bicarbonate ions

Bicarbonate ions do not easily move across the renal cell membranes, so direct reabsorption of the bicarbonate ions within the ultrafiltrate does not occur. Bicarbonate ions are instead reabsorbed through a reaction in the tubules between the filtered bicarbonate ions and the hydrogen ions, which are secreted by the tubular cells. H_2CO_3 is formed, and then disassociates into CO_2 and H_2O.

The CO_2 immediately diffuses back across the cell membrane and recombines with H_2O under the influence of carbonic anhydrase, thereby generating more H_2CO_3. The H_2CO_3 disassociates to form a hydrogen ion and a bicarbonate ion: the bicarbonate diffuses across the cell membrane into the interstitial fluid and then the peritubular capillaries into blood. Therefore, each time a hydrogen ion is formed in the tubular epithelial cells, a bicarbonate ion is also formed and released into the blood (McGloin & McLeod 2010).

If bicarbonate ions exceed hydrogen ions in the filtrate, the excess bicarbonate is excreted, as it cannot be reabsorbed. This helps to correct a potential metabolic alkalosis. If a metabolic acidosis occurs, the excess amount of hydrogen allows for all the bicarbonate to be reabsorbed, and any remaining hydrogen is excreted in the urine.

Hydrogen ion secretion is therefore necessary – both for bicarbonate reabsorption and the manufacturing of new bicarbonate. Under normal conditions, the tubules must secrete enough hydrogen to ensure that all the bicarbonate is reabsorbed. During an alkalosis, hydrogen secretion is reduced to enable excretion of bicarbonate. Conversely, during an acidosis, hydrogen ion secretion is increased to promote the amount of bicarbonate within the blood. There are two important stimuli for increasing hydrogen ion secretion during acidosis. These are: an increase in the pCO_2 of the extracellular fluid; and an increase in the hydrogen ion concentration of the extracellular fluid. In addition, aldosterone stimulates hydrogen ion secretion by the intercalated cells (McGloin & McLeod 2010).

Test yourself

What is an acid?

What is a base?

What are the three mechanisms to maintain acid-base balance?

What substances are examples of buffers?

What is the respiratory response?

What is the renal response?

Interpreting blood gases

Interpreting arterial blood gases accurately is an essential part of caring for a patient who is critically ill or displaying signs of acute deterioration. When interpreting blood gases, a systematic approach will help determine whether or not the pH is altered, and whether this change is due to an acidosis or an alkalosis. In addition, the practitioner needs to identify whether any alterations are due to a respiratory or metabolic cause. If these changes are chronic or long-term, the body will endeavour to maintain a normal pH for the cellular activity so compensation may be demonstrated.

Respiratory disturbances

Table 4.1 Causes of respiratory disturbances in arterial blood gases

Respiratory acidosis	**Respiratory alkalosis**
• Airway obstruction • Mechanical ventilation leading to hypercarbia • Neuromuscular causes (e.g. Guillain–Barré syndrome, myasthenia gravis, motor neurone disease) • Central nervous system causes (e.g. head injury, cerebral infections) • Sedatives and narcotic drugs • Decreased chest wall compliance (e.g. pneumothorax, abdominal distension, burns) • Loss of chest wall integrity (e.g. flail segment) • Increased small airways resistance (e.g. asthma) • Decreased lung compliance (e.g. acute respiratory distress syndrome, pneumonia, pulmonary oedema)	**Acute:** • Hypoxaemia • Liver failure • Sepsis • Asthma • Opiate or benzodiazepine withdrawal • Mechanical hyperventilation • Pain • Anxiety **Chronic:** • Pregnancy • Chronic lung disease • High altitude

If the alteration has a respiratory cause, the *primary* change will be in the carbon dioxide level. Carbon dioxide can be classed as an acid. Therefore, if there is an increase in carbon dioxide, the pH drops and the patient is said to have a respiratory acidosis. The reverse will happen if there is a decrease in the carbon dioxide, and the patient will be said to have a respiratory alkalosis (Bersten & Soni 2014).

The primary cause of a respiratory acidosis is usually hypoventilation. Conditions that can lead to hypoventilation include: a decreased level of consciousness, a reduction in neuromuscular function, chronic respiratory dysfunction and musculoskeletal disorders. In contrast, respiratory alkalosis is commonly caused by hyperventilation, which can occur if someone is anxious or in pain (see Table 4.1). Respiratory alkalosis can also occur in pregnancy, liver failure, asthma and when withdrawing from opiates or benzodiazepines (Bersten & Soni 2014).

Metabolic disturbances

Table 4.2 Causes of metabolic disturbances in arterial blood gases

Metabolic acidosis	**Metabolic alkalosis**
• Lactate acidosis • Ketoacidosis • Renal failure or acute kidney injury • Salicylate overdose • Large volumes of saline infusion • Diarrhoea	• Loop or thiazide diuretics • Cushing's syndrome • Mineralocorticosteroid excess • Hypercalacaemia • Magnesium deficiency **Loss of acid:** • Vomiting or loss of gastric fluid • Laxative abuse **Gain of alkaline:** • Sodium bicarbonate administration • Sodium citrate administration (e.g. in massive blood transfusion) • Renal replacement

When alterations in pH have a metabolic cause, the *primary* change will be in the bicarbonate level. Bicarbonate is an alkaline substance so if there is an increase in the bicarbonate level, there will be an increase in the pH. A metabolic alkalosis is therefore seen. If there is a decrease in bicarbonate levels, a metabolic acidosis occurs.

With metabolic changes, it is important to determine whether the alteration is due to a loss or gain of an alkalotic or acidic substance. For instance, a metabolic alkalosis could either be due to a gain of alkaline substances (such as ingestion of antacids) or to a loss of acid (which could occur with vomiting). Conversely, metabolic acidosis can be caused by loss of alkaline substances (for example, during diarrhoea). It can also result from an increase in acid in the blood (which can occur with acute kidney injury) and poor cellular perfusion due to hypotension or hypovolaemia (see Table 4.2).

Mixed gases

Sometimes the blood gas may show both respiratory and metabolic causes for the change in pH. These cases are known as mixed disorders. In a mixed acidosis, the drop in pH is caused by both a high pCO_2 and a low HCO_3. This can happen, for example, following a cardiac arrest when there has been a period of hypoventilation and reduced perfusion. A mixed alkalosis is demonstrated by a high pH, a low pCO_2 and a high HCO_3. This can occur, for example, with liver dysfunction.

Compensatory mechanisms

In certain situations, when there has been ongoing derangement of values, compensation is seen in the blood gas results. This can be partial compensation (when the pH is still abnormal) or full compensation, when the pH is within a normal range despite pCO_2 and HCO_3 measurements that are outside normal limits.

In compensation, the primary cause will be compensated for by the 'opposite' system. For example, with chronic carbon dioxide retention (which may be seen in a patient with chronic obstructive pulmonary disease), the high levels of carbon dioxide are compensated for by retention of bicarbonate. Therefore, there is metabolic compensation for the respiratory problem.

In metabolic acidosis, the compensation will be a reduction in carbon dioxide, resulting from an increase in respiratory rate. Carbon dioxide is removed, to compensate for the metabolic acidosis, and the pH is thus helped to return to a normal range. This explains why tachypnoea (abnormally deep breathing) is seen in shock situations (McGloin & McLeod 2010). The limiting factor to this response is the amount of bicarbonate available to buffer the hydrogen.

Blood gas analysis

As we have seen, the first step in analysing and interpreting blood gases is to look at the pH and determine whether the pH is normal, high (alkalosis) or low (acidosis). Following this, primary changes in the pCO_2 or the HCO_3 need to be identified so that the source of the change in pH can be identified. This enables practitioners to determine whether the change in pH is respiratory or metabolic in origin. There are some situations where the change in pH can be due to both respiratory and metabolic causes – that is, a mixed acidosis or alkalosis. The final step is to observe for compensation and, if this is present, find out whether there is full or partial compensation. Any hypoxaemia will be reflected in the pO_2. However, the pO_2 will not directly alter the pH (see Figure 4.1).

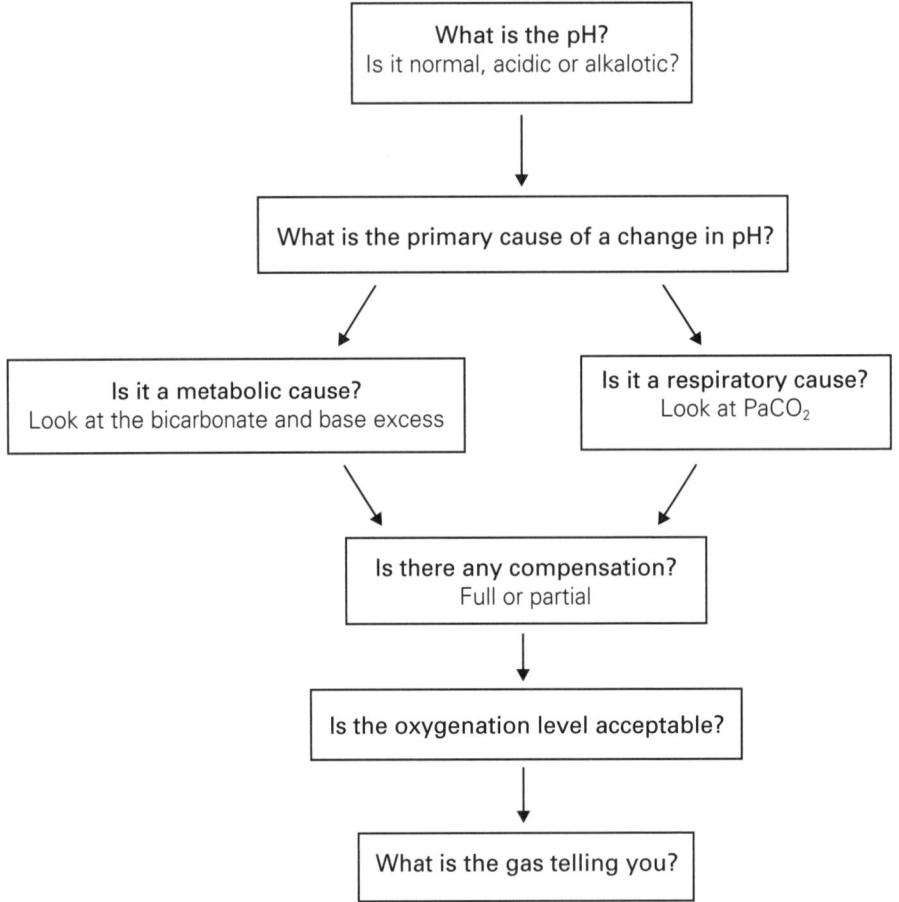

Figure 4.1 Steps in interpreting blood gases

By remembering normal ranges for each parameter, and considering whether they are normal, above normal range or below, the blood gases can easily be interpreted (see Table 4.3).

Table 4.3 Interpretation of arterial blood gases

	pH	pCO$_2$	HCO$_3$	BE
Respiratory acidosis	Reduced	Increased	Normal	Normal
Respiratory alkalosis	Increased	Reduced	Normal	Normal
Metabolic acidosis	Reduced	Normal	Reduced	Reduced
Metabolic alkalosis	Increased	Normal	Increased	Increased
Respiratory acidosis with partial metabolic compensation	Reduced	Increased	Increased	Increased
Metabolic acidosis with partial respiratory compensation	Reduced	Reduced	Reduced	Reduced
Mixed acidosis	Reduced	Increased	Reduced	Reduced
Mixed alkalosis	Increased	Reduced	Increased	Increased
Fully compensated	Normal	Increased	Increased	Increased

Test yourself

Using Figure 4.1 and Table 4.3, try to interpret these blood gases.

1) pH 7.33
   PaO$_2$ 11kPa
   PaCO$_2$ 6.3kPa
   HCO$_3$ 24mmol/l
   BE 0

2) pH 7.37
   PaO$_2$ 8kPa
   PaCO$_2$ 4.8kPa
   HCO$_3$ 22mmol/l
   BE -1

3) pH 7.47
   PaO_2 12kPa
   $PaCO_2$ 5.2kPa
   HCO_3 28mmol/l
   BE +4

4) pH 7.32
   PaO_2 9kPa
   $PaCO_2$ 5.2kPa
   HCO_3 18mmol/l
   BE -5

5) pH 7.5
   PaO_2 10kPa
   $PaCO_2$ 4.2kPa
   HCO_3 24mmol/l
   BE 1

6) pH 7.31
   PaO_2 12kPa
   $PaCO_2$ 4.0kPa
   HCO_3 17mmol/l
   BE -5

7) pH 7.33
   PaO_2 8kPa
   $PaCO_2$ 7.2kPa
   HCO_3 28mmol/l
   BE +6

8) pH   7.44
   PaO_2 9kPa
   $PaCO_2$ 7.0kPa
   HCO_3 29mmol/l
   BE   +7

9) pH   7.1
   PaO_2 7kPa
   $PaCO_2$ 7.5kPa
   HCO_3 12mmol/l
   BE   -10

10) pH   7.5
    PaO_2 13kPa
    $PaCO_2$ 3.7kPa
    HCO_3 28mmol/l
    BE   +6

5

How to respond to the results

Once any changes in the blood gases have been correctly identified, appropriate adjustments to patient management can be considered. When deciding on changes in interventions, the patient's underlying condition and the overall aims of their care must be taken into account. This will ensure that the changes made are relevant and appropriate to the individual patient's situation.

Reduced PaO_2
Self-ventilating patients

A low PaO_2 is an indication of hypoxaemia, which can result in reduced tissue perfusion. This may manifest as organ dysfunction (such as confusion) and can contribute to the production of lactate. Lactate is a by-product of anaerobic cellular respiration and is a sign of reduced perfusion. Cells are unable to break down glucose by using oxygen, as they would normally do (McGloin & McLeod 2010).

If there is a reduction in PaO_2, supplementary oxygen needs to be commenced in order to achieve a PaO_2 that is appropriate for that patient. Fixed rate oxygen devices (such as venturi systems) may be useful in situations where there is concern about the PaO_2, as they ensure that the prescribed percentage of oxygen is delivered regardless of the depth of breathing.

Should higher concentrations of oxygen be insufficient to improve the pO_2, continuous positive airway pressure (CPAP) may be commenced. CPAP delivers oxygen under positive pressure throughout the respiratory breath cycle (Marino 2014). The application of the positive pressure means that the alveoli remain open at the end of expiration. This increases the functional residual capacity, which enhances gas exchange. In addition, the work of breathing is reduced, as there is an improvement in lung compliance (Marino 2014).

The CPAP circuit consists of a flow generator that can deliver oxygen under positive pressure, a tightly fitting mask and a CPAP valve (or flow resistor) in the distal portion of the circuit, through which the patient exhales. There needs to be enough pressure from the flow generator to keep the valve in the flow resistor open throughout inhalation and exhalation. This indicates that the alveoli are also open throughout the breath cycle. Usually, there is a second CPAP valve in the circuit, which requires a higher pressure to open it. This valve is a safety mechanism: the patient will be able to breathe through it if the other valve fails to open properly.

The CPAP mask needs to be tight fitting to avoid leakage; and patients may find this difficult to tolerate, especially if they feel claustrophobic. Pressure damage may develop and any air leaks could cause corneal dryness and abrasions. Therefore, CPAP via face mask is used as a temporary measure to avoid or postpone intubation (Marino 2014).

CPAP via face mask cannot be used with patients who have a reduced level of consciousness, as there is a risk they may aspirate. Further contraindications are: a pneumothorax, significant hypotension and head or facial trauma. The raised intrathoracic pressures can worsen any pneumothorax and may also reduce cardiac output, which will worsen any hypotension. The tight mask and straps can reduce cerebral venous return and could therefore increase intracranial pressure. In the case of facial fractures, the application of the mask will not only be painful but could put the patient at risk of developing a pneumocele.

CPAP helmets are also being used in the critical care setting. These avoid some of the complications of using a CPAP mask and are generally less claustrophobic and better tolerated (Antonelli *et al.* 2005). The transparent helmet allows for better patient communication and interaction with their surroundings.

Mechanically ventilated patients

If the patient is being mechanically ventilated and has a hypoxaemia, altering the fraction of inspired oxygen (F_iO_2) can help to improve the PaO_2, as can increasing the positive end expiratory pressure (PEEP), which is similar to CPAP. If these actions do not resolve the hypoxaemia, the inspired–expired ratio (I:E) ratio can be changed to lengthen the inspiratory time, which can also improve oxygen delivery.

Alterations in $PaCO_2$

Respiratory acidosis (increased $PaCO_2$)

A respiratory acidosis develops when there is hypoventilation. This can be due to a variety of reasons but the aim of treatment is to increase the expired minute volume. Therefore the respiratory rate and/or tidal volume (size of breath) need to be increased; how this is achieved will depend on the patient's particular situation.

If there is a reduced level of consciousness leading to hypoventilation and retention of carbon dioxide (for example, due to sedation, analgesics or recreational drugs), reversal agents to the drug may be administered. This action should result in an improved level of consciousness, with a subsequent increase in respiratory rate and resolution of the hypoventilation. As the respiratory rate increases, the pH of the blood should normalise as the $PaCO_2$ reduces to a normal level.

Mechanical ventilation may be required if the respiratory acidosis is due to reasons other than sedation or analgesics, or if the effect of the drugs persists.

Non-invasive ventilation (NIV)

NIV can offer an easier alternative to invasive ventilatory support and the British Thoracic Society (2002) recommends that NIV is indicated for situations including: COPD with a respiratory acidosis, hypercapnic respiratory failure secondary to neuromuscular disease – for example, Guillain-Barré syndrome, myasthenia gravis or spinal injuries, or chest wall deformity, such as scoliosis.

The principle of NIV is to reduce carbon dioxide by increasing the patient's spontaneous minute volume. During NIV, there is alternation between two pressure levels during breathing: a higher level on inspiration and a lower one on expiration (McGloin & McLeod 2010). The inspiratory positive airway pressure (IPAP) provides extra support on inspiration so that a larger inspiratory tidal volume is taken. IPAP also reduces the work of breathing and increases alveolar ventilation (Tully 2002).

The expiratory positive airway pressure (EPAP) helps to prevent alveolar collapse in a similar way to CPAP and increases functional residual capacity. Larger volumes enter and leave the lungs, thereby improving carbon dioxide clearance. Increasing the difference between the IPAP and the EPAP increases the pressure support for the breath, thus further enhancing further carbon dioxide clearance if required (McGloin & McLeod 2010).

The primary aim of NIV is to improve carbon dioxide levels. However, oxygen can also be administered with NIV should a hypoxaemia be evident. Like CPAP, NIV is usually delivered via a tight-fitting mask. Therefore the same complications of the mask apply. Also, similarly to CPAP, NIV cannot be used if the patient has a reduced level of consciousness.

Invasive ventilation

Invasive ventilation requires either an endotracheal tube or a tracheostomy to support respiratory function. Mechanical ventilation creates lung expansion by forcing the lungs to inflate through the application of positive pressure (Adam & Osborne 2005). This can be achieved by delivering a set volume for each mechanical breath (volume cycled ventilation) or by identifying a pressure up to which the ventilator will deliver gas flow (pressure cycled ventilation). In pressure cycled ventilation, the pressure set in combination with the patient's lung compliance determines the tidal volume delivered (McGloin & McLeod 2010).

If a patient has a respiratory acidosis (or the $PaCO_2$ is higher than desired), the mechanical respiratory rate can be manipulated, as can the tidal volumes for each breath. Both these actions will enhance the expired minute volume, which controls expired carbon dioxide. Therefore, if using a ventilation mode such as synchronised intermittent volume cycled ventilation with volume control (SIMV (VC)), the $PaCO_2$ can be easily reduced by increasing the respiratory rate or tidal volume. However, if using a mode such as SIMV with pressure control (SIMV (PC)), to reduce the $PaCO_2$, the respiratory rate can be increased or the upper pressure limit can be raised so that a bigger tidal volume is delivered from the ventilator.

Respiratory alkalosis (reduced $PaCO_2$)

The primary cause of respiratory alkalosis is hyperventilation. Irrespective of whether the patient is self ventilating or mechanically ventilated, it is important to reduce the expired minute volume and this is usually achieved by reducing the respiratory rate.

If the patient is self ventilating, the underlying cause must be identified and addressed. Therefore, if the patient is in pain, analgesics should be offered. Or if the patient is very anxious, reassurance will help. If necessary, the use of a rebreathe system may be required, in which the patient breathes back their expired carbon dioxide to increase their $PaCO_2$. This is useful when someone is hyperventilating – during a panic attack, for example.

If the patient is mechanically ventilated, the minute volume needs to be reduced. This can be achieved by reducing the mechanical respiratory rate or the tidal volume. If the patient is on pressure-cycled ventilation, the upper pressure can be reduced so that a smaller tidal volume is delivered (McGloin & McLeod 2010).

Alterations in bicarbonate and base excess
Metabolic acidosis (reduced HCO_3^- and BE)

In the case of a metabolic acidosis, it is important to identify and treat the underlying cause (Bersten & Soni 2015). It is therefore imperative to start by considering whether the acidosis has developed due to a gain of hydrogen ions or due to a loss of bicarbonate. Knowledge of the patient and their underlying condition will help determine this.

One of the common causes of a gain of hydrogen ions is shock. As there is reduced cardiac output and perfusion to cells during shock, the cells start to undergo anaerobic respiration, with subsequent production of lactate and hydrogen as by-products. This can create a metabolic acidosis, and fluid resuscitation will help to restore perfusion.

Acute kidney injury (AKI) can also lead to a metabolic acidosis, as hydrogen cannot be effectively cleared from the blood. First-line renal management aims to restore perfusion to the kidneys and this can help in blood clearance of hydrogen. However, if fluid resuscitation and blood support is insufficient to resolve the acidosis, renal replacement therapy may be required to help to restore a normal pH (McGloin & McLeod 2010).

With significant metabolic acidosis, the administration of alkalinising drugs (such as sodium bicarbonate) may be considered. This strategy is largely supported for metabolic acidosis due to loss of bicarbonate (as may be seen with severe diarrhoea), rather than lactic acidosis (Adeva-Andany *et al.* 2014). Dellinger *et al.* (2013) do not recommend the use of bicarbonate in septic patients with hypoperfusion-induced lactic acidosis, with a pH ≥7.15. In addition, the current resuscitation guidelines do not recommend the routine use of bicarbonate during cardiopulmonary resuscitation (Resuscitation Council 2010).

Metabolic alkalosis (increased HCO_3^- and BE)

As with metabolic acidosis, it is important to start by identifying and removing the cause. Diuretic therapy may need to be altered if this is the underlying cause. Alternatively, electrolyte replacement, such as potassium, may be required, as may renal replacement therapy (see Table 5.1).

Table 5.1 Actions to take to resolve changes in arterial blood gases

	Action
Respiratory acidosis	**Increase expired minute volume** ● Increase respiratory rate ● Increase tidal volume (if on NIV or pressure- cycled invasive ventilation, increase the IPAP or pressure control level)
Respiratory alkalosis	**Decrease expired ventilation** If self ventilating: ● Identify cause ● Rebreathing may be required. If mechanically ventilated: ● Reduce respiratory rate ● Reduce tidal volume.

Metabolic acidosis	**Treat cause** ● If in shock, may require fluid resuscitation or blood pressure support ● If acute kidney injury is evident, renal replacement may be required.
Metabolic alkalosis	**Treat cause** ● Consider diuretics and electrolyte replacement ● Renal replacement may be required.
Respiratory acidosis with partial metabolic compensation	**Treat original cause**
Metabolic acidosis with partial respiratory compensation	**Treat original cause**
Fully compensated	**Leave**

When compensation is present, care needs to be taken to avoid an abrupt change in pH. For example, if the patient has a metabolic acidosis with respiratory compensation, commencing mechanical ventilation could alter the $PaCO_2$ rapidly if a 'normal' pCO_2 is achieved, which could then further reduce the pH. This could be lethal. Similarly, if a patient normally retains carbon dioxide and has compensated for this, commencing NIV or mechanical ventilation may result in a metabolic alkalosis as the carbon dioxide is removed, leaving a high bicarbonate or base excess.

How to respond to the results

Test yourself

With each blood gas listed in Chapter 4, identify what actions could be undertaken to resolve any abnormalities in the blood gases.

Case study 1: Simon

You are looking after Simon who has returned to the critical care unit following cardiac surgery. He is still intubated and ventilated on a volume-cycled mode. He has been cardiovascularly stable since return and is starting to warm up following the surgery.

His initial observations are:

HR	85BPM
BP	110/60mmHg
MAP	76mmHg
CVP	7mmHg
Temperature	35.7°C

Ventilator observations:

RR	12BPM
Tidal volumes	380ml (5ml/kg ideal body weight)
PEEP	5cm H_2O
Airway pressures	+18cm H_2O

Arterial blood gases:

pH	7.34
PaO_2	11kPa
$PaCO_2$	5.2kPa
HCO_3	22mmol/l
BE	-1mmol/l

His observations 30 minutes later are:

HR	95BPM
BP	105/50mmHg
MAP	68mmHg
CVP	7mmHg
Temperature	36.4°C

Arterial Blood Gas Analysis – making it easy

Ventilator observations:

RR 12BPM
Tidal volumes 380ml (5ml/kg ideal body weight)
PEEP 5cm H_2O
Airway pressures +18cm H_2O

Arterial blood gases:

pH 7.33
PaO_2 11kPa
$PaCO_2$ 5.2kPa
HCO_3 18mmol/l
BE -3mmol/l

a) How would you interpret these blood gases?

b) What do you think has caused the changes?

c) What actions do you think should be taken?

Case study 2: Mary

You are looking after Mary who has been admitted with atypical pneumonia. She is currently self ventilating, although she is looking distressed and exhausted.

Her last set of blood gases were taken in the emergency department and showed:

pH 7.47
PaO_2 8kPa
$PaCO_2$ 4.2kPa
HCO_3 24mmol/l
BE 0mmol/l

On admission to critical care, her observations are:

HR 110BPM
BP 150/90mmHg
MAP 110mmHg
CVP 6mmHg
Temperature 38.7°C

How to respond to the results

Respiratory observations:
RR   26BPM, using accessory muscles and shallow breaths
SpO_2 88% (on non-rebreathe system)

Arterial blood gases:
pH   7.3
PaO_2 6kPa
$PaCO_2$ 6.5kPa
HCO_3 22mmol/l
BE   -1mmol/l

She is becoming drowsy and looks exhausted.

a) How would you interpret these blood gases?
b) What do you think has caused the changes?
c) What actions do you think should be taken?
d) What concerns would you have when mechanical ventilation is commenced?

Case study 3: John

You are looking after John who has just been brought to the emergency department. He has a history of COPD and he is normally on home oxygen. He has developed a chest infection.

On assessment, you find:
HR   110BPM
BP   160/90mmHg
MAP   113mmHg
Temperature   38.4°C

Respiratory observations:
RR   28BPM, using accessory muscles and shallow breaths
SpO_2 84%

Arterial blood gases:
pH   7.38
PaO_2 7kPa

PaCO$_2$ 8.5kPa
HCO$_3$ 28mmol/l
BE   +4mmol/l

When you check his blood gases 30 minutes later, they are:
pH   7.33
PaO$_2$ 6kPa
PaCO$_2$ 9.0kPa
HCO$_3$ 28mmol/l
BE   +4mmol/l

It is decided to commence non-invasive ventilation with the setting of IPAP +16 EPAP +5 with 4 litres of oxygen. *When you check his blood gases 30 minutes after commencing this non-invasive ventilation, they are:*
pH   7.34
PaO$_2$ 7kPa
PaCO$_2$ 8.8kPa
HCO$_3$ 28mmol/l
BE   +4mmol/l

a) How would you interpret these blood gases?
b) What do you think has caused the changes?
c) What actions do you think should be taken?

6

Caring for a patient with an arterial line

In patients who are critically ill or who require frequent blood gas measurement, an in-dwelling arterial line may be inserted. From this, arterial blood samples can be obtained; and if the arterial line is connected to a transducer, both the arterial blood pressure and the arterial pressure waveform can be visualised on the bedside monitor (Adam & Osborne 2005). This is helpful in patients who are haemodynamically unstable and require vasoactive drugs (such as noradrenaline or dobutamine) to support their blood pressure. In such a situation, the patient may need to be transferred to a higher dependency or intensive care setting, for advanced monitoring and support.

Arterial line sites

The radial, femoral, dorsalis pedis and brachial arteries can all be used to site arterial lines.

Radial artery

This is the preferred site, as the hand has good collateral circulation. The site is easy to observe and the artery is close to the surface of the skin, making it relatively easy to insert the line. Prior to insertion, the collateral circulation can be assessed by performing an Allen's test. To do this, both the ulnar and radial arteries are manually occluded. The patient is asked to flex their fingers, which should lead to blanching of the palm (see Figures 6.1 and 6.2, page 42).

The pressure on the ulnar artery is then released, which should lead to the palm of the hand becoming flushed (see Figure 6.3, page 43).

This demonstrates that the hand has good collateral circulation. If the patient has Raynaud's disease or poor ulnar or peripheral circulation, radial artery cannulation should be avoided, as there will be a risk of hand ischaemia, radial nerve damage and skin necrosis. Thrombosis can also develop.

Arterial Blood Gas Analysis – making it easy

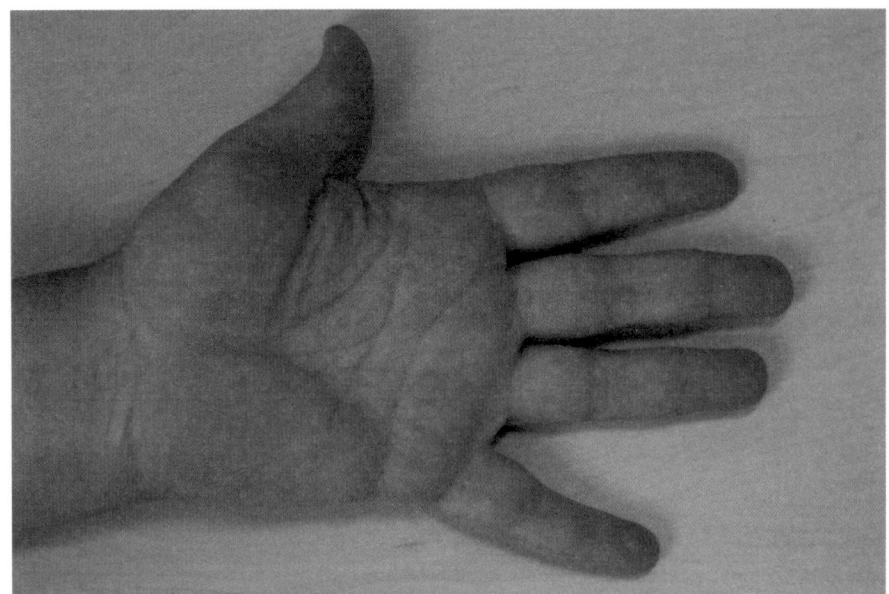

Figure 6.1 The patient's hand before starting an Allen's test

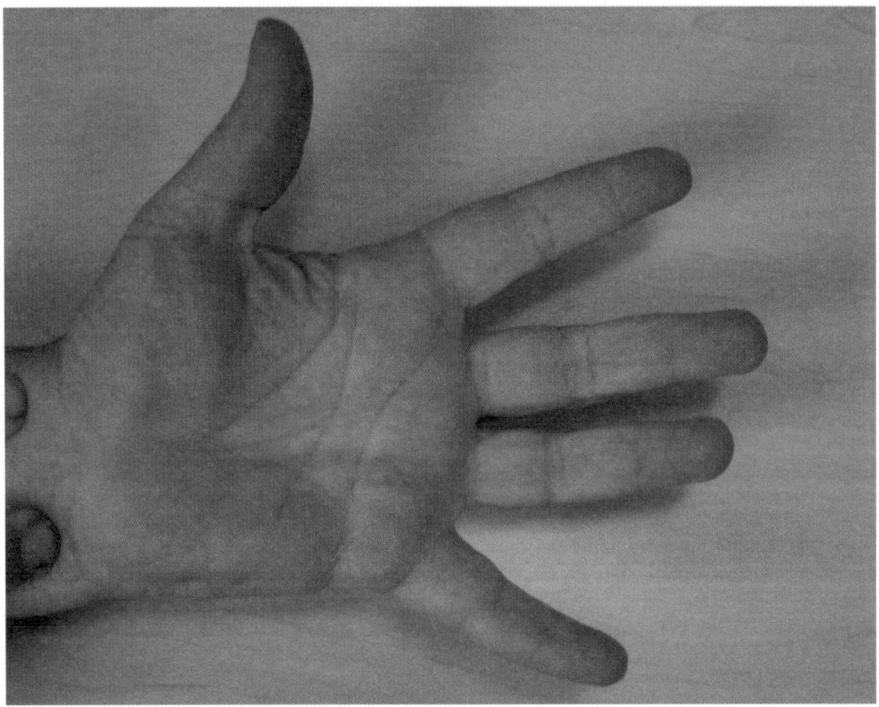

Figure 6.2 Blanching of the palm during occlusion of the ulnar and radial arteries

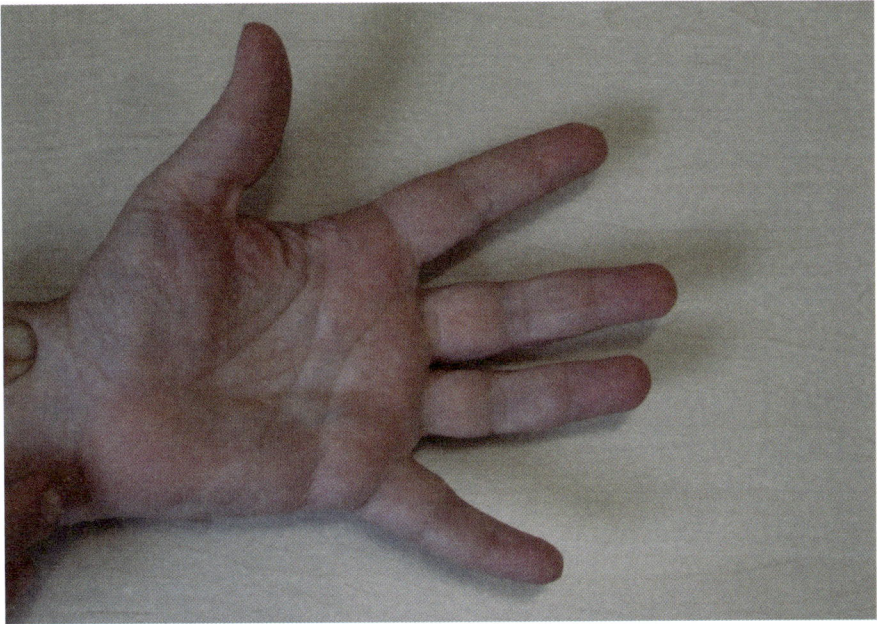

Figure 6.3 Flushing of the palm after the ulnar artery has been released, demonstrating good collateral circulation

Femoral artery

This is sometimes used in patients who are very hypotensive, as it may still be palpable and it is fairly superficial. However, if the patient has peripheral vascular disease or there is compromised blood flow to the limb, they may be at risk of developing limb ischaemia (Adam & Osborne 2005). Pedal pulses and capillary refill or tissue perfusion should therefore be frequently assessed. The site is also difficult to observe continually, so haemorrhage and line disconnection could occur and not be immediately noticed.

Dorsalis pedis artery

This site can be used but it is a small artery and can be difficult to cannulate. Using this site can restrict patient movement. It may also be difficult to obtain an accurate waveform if it is being used for arterial blood pressure monitoring. This site should be avoided if the patient has peripheral vascular disease or if they are diabetic. It is important to check the toes for any signs of ischaemia.

Brachial artery

This site should ideally be avoided and is usually only used if no other site can be cannulated. There is a risk of losing blood supply to the forearm, as it is an end artery. Therefore if the line becomes occluded, there is no alternative arterial blood supply to the forearm (Adam & Osborne 2005). If this site is used, frequent assessment of the radial pulse and limb perfusion is essential. This site reduces patient mobility, as they need to avoid bending their arm at the elbow.

Choosing a site for arterial cannulation

According to Adam and Osborne (2005), if arterial cannulation is required, the site chosen should:

- Have a good collateral blood supply so that the blood flow to the limb distal to the arterial line does not become compromised
- Not be in a limb with peripheral vascular disease or a fistula
- Be easily observable so that any disconnection or haemorrhage is noted immediately
- Not be in an area that is at risk of bacterial contamination or where there is a wound.

Safety considerations

There are six main safety considerations when inserting an arterial line:

1. Potential for haemorrhage or haematoma
2. Accidental intra-arterial injection of drugs
3. Infection at the line site
4. Risk of embolisation
5. Risk of spasm of the artery
6. Risk of thrombosis.

1. Potential for haemorrhage or haematoma

- The cannula needs to be secured with, for example, wound closure strips to avoid the risk of accidental de-cannulation (see Figure 6.4).
- A transparent occlusive dressing should be used so that the site is easily observable.
- As far as possible, the cannula site should be visible and not covered by bed linen.
- Any three-way taps in the transducer circuit should be turned off towards the atmosphere at all times (see Figure 6.5).

2. Accidental intra-arterial injection of drugs

- The arterial cannula should be clearly labelled to indicate that it is an arterial line, not a venous line.
- All staff need to be aware that no IV infusions or drugs should be administered via an arterial line.

What are arterial blood gases

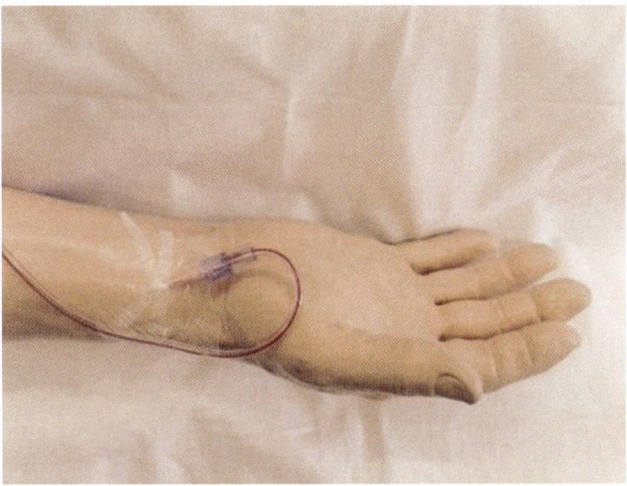

Figure 6.4 Arterial line dressing

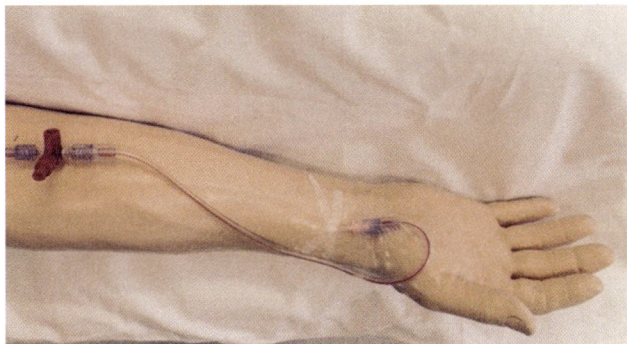

Figure 6.5 Correct arterial line set-up

3. Infection at the line site
- Asepsis should be maintained during cannulation and when priming the transducer set.
- Dressings should be changed using aseptic technique.
- Sterile bungs must be used at the three-way taps.
- Blood samples must be taken according to local policy, using aseptic technique.

4. Risk of embolisation
- All connections must be tight.
- There must be adequate flush solution connected to the transducer line and the bag must be under a pressure of 300mmHg.
- All air bubbles must be removed during priming of the transducer set.

5. Risk of spasm of the artery (this can lead to inadequate blood flow to the limb)

- The flush solution should be at room temperature.
- The cannula must not be excessively flushed.
- Assess the distal portion of the limb – if there is blanching, coolness and/or pain, the arterial line should be removed.

6. Risk of thrombosis formation

- The bag of flush solution should be at 300mmHg.
- Ensure that there is adequate fluid in the bag.

Arterial pressure monitoring

If using an in-dwelling arterial line, the arterial pressure can be transduced onto the bedside monitor so that the pressure can be continuously monitored and the pressure observed. The arterial blood pressure waveform comprises an upstroke signifying systole (the anacrotic rise), followed by a downstroke when diastole occurs. There should be a notch within the diastole limb of the waveform: this is the dicrotic notch and it occurs when the aortic valve closes (see Figure 6.6).

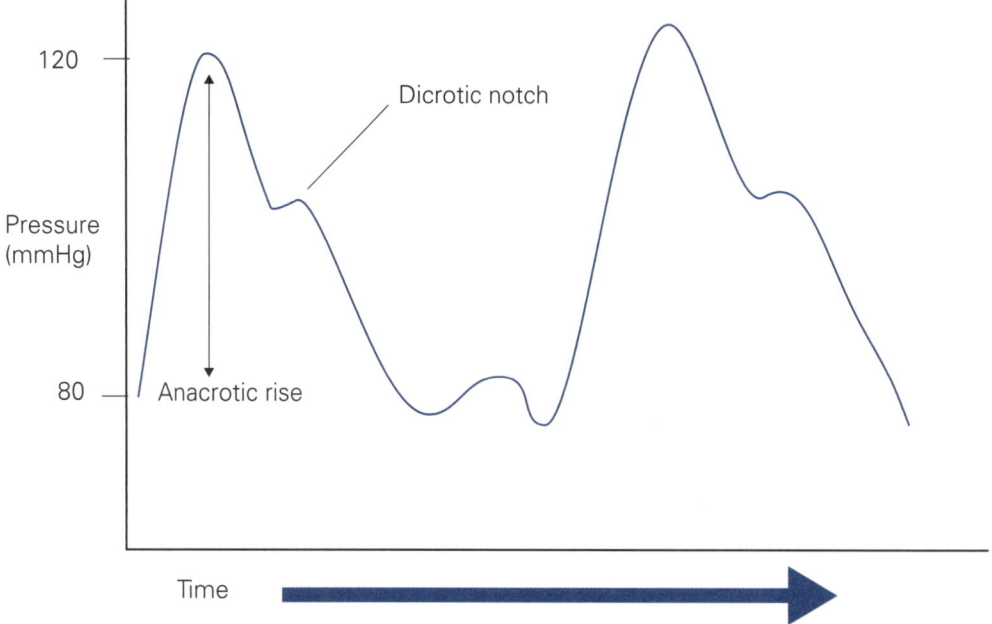

Figure 6.6 Normal arterial waveform

What are arterial blood gases

It is important that the waveform is accurate and not dampened, as this can give an inaccurate blood pressure. In an underdamp waveform, the upstroke ends in an overshoot spike, followed by multiple small spikes on the downstroke. This is called 'ringing'. It is an over-exaggerated response because of a reduced natural frequency of the fluid-filled system. This response can occur if the extension tubing is too compliant or too long, in which case the systolic pressure will be overestimated (see Figure 6.7).

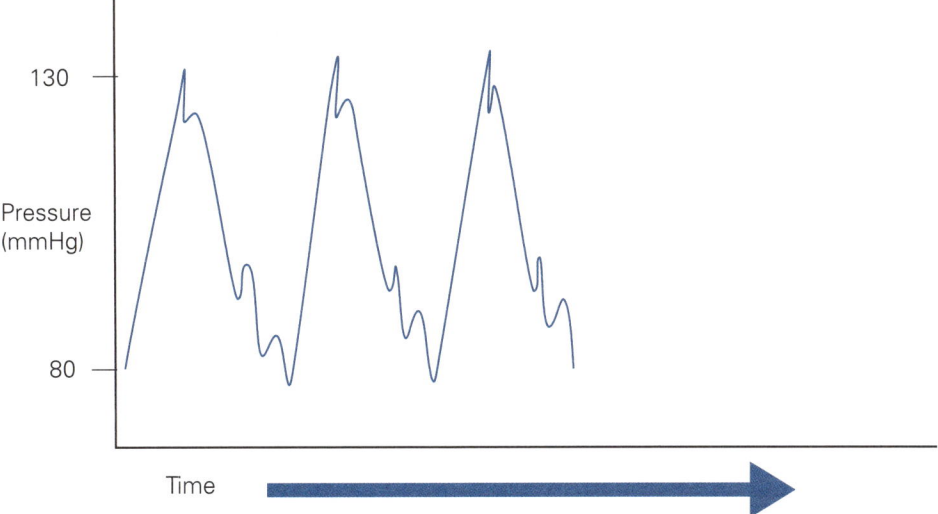

Figure 6.7 Underdamp arterial waveform

In an overdamp waveform, the waveform is indistinct, the systolic pressure is underestimated, the diastolic pressure is overestimated and the dicrotic notch may not be visible. This type of waveform is caused by air bubbles in the system, a partially obstructed catheter or extension tubing that is too long or compliant (see Figure 6.8).

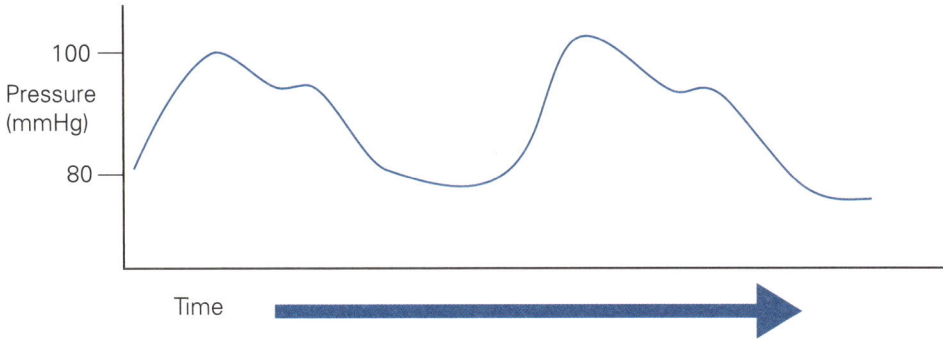

Figure 6.8 Overdamp arterial waveform

To avoid inaccurate waveforms, the arterial line transducer should be zeroed to atmospheric pressure and should be in line with the fourth intercostal space, mid axilla. This is called the phlebostatic axis. There should not be any air bubbles in the transducer line. Low compliant tubing should be used, and the addition of further tubing should be avoided. In addition, the flush fluid should be maintained at a pressure of 300mmHg and kinking or blockage of the arterial line should be avoided. As required, the arterial line can be flushed using the flush device within the transducer line. However, arterial lines should not be manually flushed, using a syringe.

Test yourself

1. What sites are commonly used for arterial line insertion?
2. Why should an Allen's test be performed prior to the insertion of a radial arterial line?
3. Identify three actions that will reduce the risk of accidental haemorrhage.
4. What can lead to an overdamp arterial waveform?
5. What actions should be undertaken to resolve an inaccurate waveform?

Test yourself answers

Chapter 1 What are arterial blood gases?

What are normal blood gas values?
pH   7.35–7.45
PaO_2 10–13.3kPa
$PaCO_2$ 4.6–6kPa
HCO_3 22–26mmol/l
BE   -2 to +2

Which ion is measured by pH?

Hydrogen

What term is used if the PaO_2 is below normal range?

Hypoxaemia

Which aspect of respiratory physiology affects $PaCO_2$?

The mechanics of respiration

Is bicarbonate an acid or alkaline substance?

Alkaline

How do buffers help to control pH?

They can remove or release hydrogen from the blood, and they act as chemical 'sponges'.

Chapter 2 Respiratory gases

What are the three key processes involved in gas exchange?

Pulmonary ventilation, external respiration, internal respiration

What is Boyle's law?

The pressure of a gas inside a container is inversely in ratio with the size of the container.

In normal respiration, does air enter the lungs under positive or negative pressure?

Negative

What key features of the alveoli–capillary membrane promote gas exchange?

Thin alveoli–capillary membrane; respiratory gases are lipid soluble which allows for easy diffusion across the cell membrane; very large surface area; good blood supply; capillaries are narrow, meaning red blood cells pass through the capillaries in single file.

By what process do respiratory gases move between the alveoli and the blood (and vice versa)?

Diffusion

What is the main influence for oxygen to disassociate from haemoglobin?

pO_2

How does a decrease in pH affect oxygen disassociation from haemoglobin?

Oxygen disassociates more easily.

What chemical formula illustrates how bicarbonate is formed from carbon dioxide?

$CO_2 + H_2O \rightarrow H_2CO_3 \rightarrow H^+ + HCO_3$ (requires carbonic anhydrase)

Chapter 3 Acid-base balance

What is an acid?

A molecule that contains hydrogen, which can be released into solutions.

What is a base?

A molecule that can combine with hydrogen.

What are the three mechanisms to maintain acid-base balance?

Buffers, respiratory response and renal response

What substances are examples of buffers?

HCO_3, phosphates, proteins and haemoglobin

What is the respiratory response?

When hydrogen combines with bicarbonate to form carbonic acid. This then splits into water and carbon dioxide, which can be expired.

Test yourself answers

What is the renal response?

Renal cells produce carbon dioxide, which combines with water to make carbonic acid, which then splits into hydrogen and bicarbonate. The bicarbonate moves into blood, whereas the hydrogen moves into the renal tubule lumen and is therefore lost in the urine.

Chapter 4 Interpreting blood gases

1) pH   7.33
   PaO_2 11kPa
   $PaCO_2$ 6.3kPa
   HCO_3 24mmol/l
   BE   0

Respiratory acidosis

2) pH   7.37
   PaO_2 8kPa
   $PaCO_2$ 4.8kPa
   HCO_3 22mmol/l
   BE   -1

Hypoxaemia; otherwise normal

3) pH   7.47
   PaO_2 12kPa
   $PaCO_2$ 5.2kPa
   HCO_3 28mmol/l
   BE   +4

Metabolic alkalosis

4) pH   7.32
   PaO_2 9kPa
   $PaCO_2$ 5.2kPa
   HCO_3 18mmol/l
   BE   -5

Metabolic acidosis; hypoxaemia

5) pH 7.5
   PaO_2 10kPa
   $PaCO_2$ 4.2kPa
   HCO_3 24mmol/l
   BE 1
Respiratory alkalosis

6) pH 7.31
   PaO_2 12kPa
   $PaCO_2$ 4.0kPa
   HCO_3 17mmol/l
   BE -5
Metabolic acidosis with partial respiratory compensation

7) pH 7.33
   PaO_2 8kPa
   $PaCO_2$ 7.2kPa
   HCO_3 28mmol/l
   BE +6
Respiratory acidosis with partial metabolic compensation; hypoxaemia

8) pH 7.44
   PaO_2 9kPa
   $PaCO_2$ 7.0kPa
   HCO_3 29mmol/l
   BE +7
Fully compensated gas; hypoxaemia

9) pH 7.1
   PaO_2 7kPa
   $PaCO_2$ 7.5kPa
   HCO_3 12mmol/l
   BE -10
Mixed acidosis; hypoxaemia

Test yourself answers

1) pH   7.5
   PaO_2 13kPa
   $PaCO_2$ 3.7kPa
   HCO_3 28mmol/l
   BE   +6

Mixed alkalosis

Chapter 5 How to respond to the results

With each blood gas listed above from Chapter 4, identify what actions could be undertaken to resolve any abnormalities in the blood gases.

1) pH   7.33
   PaO_2 11kPa
   $PaCO_2$ 6.3kPa
   HCO_3 24mmol/l
   BE   0

Increase expired minute volume.

2) pH   7.37
   PaO_2 8kPa
   $PaCO_2$ 4.8kPa
   HCO_3 22mmol/l
   BE   -1

Increase inspired oxygen.

3) pH   7.47
   PaO_2 12kPa
   $PaCO_2$ 5.2kPa
   HCO_3 28mmol/l
   BE   +4

Identify cause and treat.

4) pH   7.32
   PaO_2 9Kpa
   $PaCO_2$ 5.2kPa

HCO₃ 18mmol/l
BE   -5

Identify cause and treat; increase inspired oxygen.

5) pH   7.5
   PaO₂ 10kPa
   PaCO₂ 4.2kPa
   HCO₃ 24mmol/l
   BE   1

Reduce expired minute volume.

6) pH   7.31
   PaO₂ 12kPa
   PaCO₂ 4.0kPa
   HCO₃ 17mmol/l
   BE   -5

Treat cause of metabolic acidosis.

7) pH   7.33
   PaO₂ 8kPa
   PaCO₂ 7.2kPa
   HCO₃ 28mmol/l
   BE   +6

Treat cause of respiratory acidosis; increase inspired oxygen if this is non-COPD in origin.

8) pH   7.44
   PaO₂ 9kPa
   PaCO₂ 7.0kPa
   HCO₃ 29mmol/l
   BE   +7

Increase inspired oxygen if non-COPD. Identify original cause.

9) pH   7.1
   PaO₂ 7kPa

Test yourself answers

PaCO$_2$ 7.5kPa
HCO$_3$ 12mmol/l
BE   -10

Resolve pCO$_2$ first; see effect on pH once pCO$_2$ is within normal limits. If acidosis continues once pCO$_2$ is normal, address metabolic acidosis.

8) pH   7.5
   PaO$_2$ 13kPa
   PaCO$_2$ 3.7kPa
   HCO$_3$ 28mmol/l
   BE   +6

Treat underlying condition.

Case study 1: Simon

You are looking after Simon who has returned to the critical care unit following cardiac surgery. He is still intubated and ventilated on a volume-cycled mode. He has been cardiovascularly stable since return and is starting to warm up following the surgery.

His initial observations are:
  HR   85BPM
  BP   110/60mmHg
  MAP   76mmHg
  CVP   7mmHg
  Temperature 35.7°C

Ventilator observations:
  RR   12BPM
  Tidal volumes   380ml (5ml/kg ideal body weight)
  PEEP   5cm H$_2$O
  Airway pressures +18cm H$_2$O

Arterial blood gases:
  pH   7.34
  PaO$_2$ 11kPa
  PaCO$_2$ 5.2kPa
  HCO$_3$ 22mmol/l
  BE   -1mmol/l

Arterial Blood Gas Analysis – making it easy

His observations 30 minutes later are:
- HR   95BPM
- BP   105/50mmHg
- MAP   68mmHg
- CVP   7mmHg
- Temperature 36.4°C

Ventilator observations:
- RR   12BPM
- Tidal volumes   380ml (5ml/kg ideal body weight)
- PEEP   5cm H_2O
- Airway pressures +18cm H_2O

Arterial blood gases:
- pH   7.33
- PaO_2 11kPa
- $PaCO_2$ 5.2kPa
- HCO_3 18mmol/l
- BE   -3mmol/l

a) How would you interpret these blood gases?
The first arterial blood gas is essentially normal. The second blood gas indicates a metabolic acidosis.

b) What do you think has caused the changes?
His blood pressure has decreased, probably due to the increase in his temperature during re-warming. This has led to a reduction in tissue perfusion, which has subsequently resulted in anaerobic cellular respiration. Hydrogen and lactate are released as by-products, thereby causing the metabolic acidosis.

c) What actions do you think should be taken?
His BP needs to be supported initially with fluids. If this does not increase his BP and control the metabolic acidosis, then a vasopressor (such as noradrenaline) may need to be commenced. Re-warming needs to be slowed down slightly.

Case study 2: Mary

You are looking after Mary who has been admitted with atypical pneumonia. She is currently self ventilating although she is looking distressed and exhausted. Her last set of blood gases were taken in the emergency

Test yourself answers

department and showed:
- pH 7.47
- PaO_2 8kPa
- $PaCO_2$ 4.2kPa
- HCO_3 24mmol/l
- BE 0mmol/l

On admission to critical care, her observations are:
- HR 110BPM
- BP 150/90mmHg
- MAP 110mmHg
- CVP 6mmHg
- Temperature 38.7°C

Respiratory observations:
- RR 26BPM, using accessory muscles and shallow breaths
- SpO_2 88% (on non-rebreathe system)

Arterial blood gases:
- pH 7.3
- PaO_2 6kPa
- $PaCO_2$ 6.5kPa
- HCO_3 22mmol/l
- BE -1mmol/l

She is becoming drowsy and looks exhausted.

a) How would you interpret these blood gases?
The first arterial blood gas indicates a respiratory alkalosis with hypoxaemia. The second blood gas indicates respiratory acidosis.

b) What do you think has caused the changes?
When the first blood gas was taken, Mary was hyperventilating – hence the reduced $PaCO_2$. The second gas suggests that she has become tired or exhausted and is now not effectively ventilating. The hypoxaemia has worsened.

c) What actions do you think should be taken?
She needs to be intubated and mechanically ventilated. NIV could be considered. However, she is becoming drowsy so there would be concerns about her ability to maintain her airway.

d) What concerns would you have when mechanical ventilation is commenced?

Her $PaCO_2$ could become very high, with a subsequent worsening in the acidosis, as her mechanical respiratory rate will be less than her spontaneous rate. She will need reasonable PEEP/increased F_iO_2 to address the hypoxaemia.

Case study 3: John

You are looking after John who has just been brought to the emergency department. He has a history of COPD and he is normally on home oxygen. He has developed a chest infection.

On assessment, you find:
- HR   110BPM
- BP   160/90mmHg
- MAP   113mmHg
- Temperature 38.4°C

Respiratory observations:
- RR   28BPM, using accessory muscles and shallow breaths
- SpO_2 84%

Arterial blood gases:
- pH   7.38
- PaO_2 7kPa
- $PaCO_2$ 8.5kPa
- HCO_3 28mmol/l
- BE   +4mmol/l

When you check his blood gases 30 minutes later, they are:
- pH   7.33
- PaO_2 6kPa
- $PaCO_2$ 9.0kPa
- HCO_3 28mmol/l
- BE   +4mmol/l

It is decided to commence non-invasive ventilation with the setting of IPAP +16 EPAP +5 with 4 litres of oxygen. When you check his blood gases 30 minutes after commencing this non-invasive ventilation, they are:
- pH   7.34
- PaO_2 7kPa
- $PaCO_2$ 8.8kPa
- HCO_3 28mmol/l
- BE   +4mmol/l

a) How would you interpret these blood gases?

The first arterial blood gas indicates a fully compensated blood gas; the second blood gas indicates a respiratory acidosis – he is now retaining more carbon dioxide than normal and has therefore become acidotic. The final blood gas shows a respiratory acidosis.

b) What do you think has caused the changes?

He is probably tiring and his ventilation has therefore worsened.

c) What actions do you think should be taken?

With the final blood gas, the NIV settings are not effectively clearing his $PaCO_2$. The IPAP needs to be increased to support his tidal volumes more. This will increase his minute volume, which will reduce his $PaCO_2$.

Chapter 6 Caring for a patient with an arterial line

1) What sites are commonly used for arterial line insertion?

Radial, brachial, femoral, dorsalis pedis

2) Why should an Allen's test be performed prior to the insertion of a radial arterial line?

To assess whether there is adequate collateral circulation via the ulnar artery, should the radial artery become occluded.

3) Identify three actions that will reduce the risk of accidental haemorrhage.

Secure the line with the use of wound closure strips and clear occlusive dressing.

Ensure all connections are tight and the three-way tap is off to the atmosphere.

Ensure that the line site (as far as possible) is visible at all times.

4) What can lead to an overdamp arterial waveform?

Partially obstructed line (kinked), air bubbles, too long tubing used, use of additional tubing which has a different compliance, empty fluid bag, pressure < 300mmHg.

5) What actions should be undertaken to resolve an inaccurate waveform?

Re-zero, check for any kinking of line (e.g. flex patient wrist), check for air bubbles, check there is enough flush fluid, ensure pressure bag is 300mmHg, gently flush line using flush device within transducer set (do not manually flush using normal saline).

References

Adam, S.K. & Osborne, S. (2005). *Critical Care Nursing: Science and Practice*. 2nd edn. Oxford: Oxford University Press.

Adeva-Andany, M., Fernández-Fernández, C., Mouriño-Bayolo, D., Castro-Quintela, E. & Domínguez-Montero, A. (2014). Sodium Bicarbonate Therapy in Patients with Metabolic Acidosis. *The Scientific World Journal*. 2014, 627673. http://dx.doi.org/10.1155/2014/627673 (accessed 9 February 2016).

Antonelli, M., Pennisi, M.A. & Montini, L. (2005)/ Clinical review: Noninvasive ventilation in the clinical setting – experience from the past 10 years. *Critical Care*. **9** (1), 98–103.

Bersten, A.D. & Soni, N. (2014). *Oh's Intensive Care Manual*. 7th edn. London: Butterworth Heinemann.

British Thoracic Society (2002). Non-invasive ventilation in acute respiratory failure. *Thorax*. **57** (3), 192–211.

Dellinger, R.P., Levy, M.M., Rhodes, A., Annane, D., Gerlach, H., Opal, S., Sevransky, J., Sprung, C., Douglas, I., Jaeschke, R., Osborn, T., Nunnally, M., Townsend, S., Reinhart, K., Kleinpell, R., Angus, D., Deutschman, C., Machado, F., Rubenfeld, G., Webb, S., Beale, R., Vincent, J.L., Moreno, R. & the Surviving Sepsis Campaign Guidelines Committee including the Pediatric Subgroup (2013). Surviving Sepsis Campaign: International guidelines for management of severe sepsis and septic shock: 2012. *Critical Care Medicine*. **41** (2), 580–637.

Hall, J.E. (2015). *Guyton and Hall Textbook of Medical Physiology*. 13th edn. London: Saunders.

Marino, P.L. (2014). *Marino's The ICU Book*. 4th edn. London: Wolters Kluwer.

McGloin, S. & McLeod, A. (2010). *Advanced Practice in Critical Care: A Case Study Approach*. Oxford: Wiley Blackwell.

Resuscitation Council (2010). *Adult Advanced Life Support*. London: Resuscitation Council UK.

Tortora, G.J. & Derrickson, B.H. (2009). *Principles of Anatomy and Physiology*. 12th edn. New York: John Wiley and Sons.

Tully, V. (2002). Non- invasive ventilation: a guide for nursing staff. *Nursing in Critical Care*. **7** (6), 296–99.

Vander, A.J., Sherman, J.H. & Luciano, D.S. (2003). *Human Physiology: The Mechanisms of Body Function*. 9th edn. London: McGraw Hill Education.

Index

acid-base balance 1, 12, 15–21
acidosis 1, 10, 19, 23
acids 15
acute kidney injury (AKI) 35
alkalosis 1, 19, 23
Allen's test 41
arterial line safety 44–46
arterial line site choice 44
arterial line sites 41
arterial pressure monitoring 46

base excess 2
bases 15
bicarbonate buffer system 17
bicarbonate ions, reabsorption and production of 21
bicarbonate 2
blood gas analysis 25
Bohr effect 10
Boyle's law 5
buffering of hydrogen ions 16

carbon dioxide 11, 12
chloride shift 12
compensatory mechanisms 25, 36
continuous positive airway pressure (CPAP) 31
CPAP contraindications 32

expiration 6
external respiration 7

gas transport 8

haemoglobin 9
hydrogen concentration 1, 16
hydrogen ion secretion 21
hypoxaemia 2

inspiration 5
internal respiration 8
interpreting blood gases 23–27
invasive ventilation 33

kidneys 19

mechanically ventilated patients 32
metabolic acidosis 34
metabolic alkalosis 35
metabolic disturbances in arterial blood gases 24
mixed gases 25

non-invasive ventilation (NIV) 33

oxygen 9
oxygen–haemoglobin dissociation curve 9

parameters 1
partial pressure of carbon dioxide 2
partial pressure of oxygen 2
pH 1, 10
phosphate buffer system 17
primary active secretion of hydrogen ions 19
proteins as buffers 17
pulmonary ventilation 5

reduced PaO_2, response to 31
renal control of acid-base balance 19
respiratory acidosis 32
respiratory alkalosis 34
respiratory disturbances in ABGs 23
respiratory regulation of acid-base balance 18
respiratory system 5

secondary secretion of hydrogen ions 20
shock 34
supplementary oxygen 31